REBOUND

REBOUND

TRAIN YOUR MIND **TO BOUNCE BACK**
STRONGER FROM SPORTS INJURIES

CARRIE JACKSON CHEADLE
AND **CINDY KUZMA**

BLOOMSBURY SPORT
LONDON • OXFORD • NEW YORK • NEW DELHI • SYDNEY

BLOOMSBURY SPORT
Bloomsbury Publishing Plc
50 Bedford Square, London, WC1B 3DP, UK
29 Earlsfort Terrace, Dublin 2, Ireland

BLOOMSBURY, BLOOMSBURY SPORT and the Diana logo are trademarks of
Bloomsbury Publishing Plc

First published in Great Britain 2019

A catalogue record for this book is available from the British Library

Library of Congress Cataloguing-in-Publication data has been applied for

ISBN: PB: 978-1-4729-6143-3; eBook: 978-1-4729-6141-9

8 10 9

Typeset in Adobe Garamond Pro by Deanta Global Publishing Services, Chennai, India
Printed and bound in Great Britain by CPI Group (UK) Ltd. Croydon, CR0 4YY

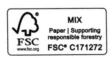

MIX
Paper | Supporting
responsible forestry
FSC® C171272

To find out more about our authors and books visit www.bloomsbury.com
and sign up for our newsletters

CONTENTS

INTRODUCTION

We're sorry you're here, but we're glad you're with us.

That's the tagline of our podcast and the virtual support group we host on Facebook, both called The Injured Athletes Club (learn more at www.injuredathletesclub.com). And it's the message we want you—the sidelined athlete—to hear, first and foremost.

If you're anything like us or the athletes we know, injury has thrown you for a loop. You're feeling sad, scared, isolated, uncertain, or all of the above. Layered on top of that might be some relief at having a break from the pressure of training or competing—followed swiftly by guilt, remorse, and yet more despair. And though you might have doctors, physical therapists or physiotherapists, and athletic trainers to guide you through the physical steps of recovery, when it comes to emotions, you might feel you're all on your own.

Until now. We're sorry you're injured—no athlete wants to be sidelined. But we're glad you found your way to these pages.

When injured athletes first meet with Carrie—a mental skills coach certified by the Association for Applied Sport Psychology—there's often a visceral, physical reaction. Carrie can see their shoulders drop, the tension in their faces relax, their eyes brighten with a glimmer of hope. *I'm not alone*, they realize. *There are others who get it. And now, I see there's a way forward.*

Over time, they learn solid, tangible skills to handle their emotions and take control of their recovery. No matter where they are in the injury and rehab process, they realize, there are ways they can optimize the situation to give themselves the best possible chance of a positive outcome.

It's our hope that this book can serve as a similar source of relief and support. Wherever you are in your injury journey, there is a way forward.

GET READY TO BOUNCE BACK

The degree to which an athlete recovers from injury varies, as does the ease with which they do so. Some of the differences have to do with factors like the severity of the setback. However, even athletes whose lives are irrevocably altered by injury often make what experts call a "remarkable recovery"—coming back mentally and physically stronger, whether they are able to return to their sport in the exact same way or not. For instance:

- Kevin Ogar, paralyzed in a weightlifting accident, now operates a fitness program for veterans, and coaches in CrossFit's adaptive program (his story's on pages 44–45)
- Carrie Tollefson overcame a cancer scare, surgery to graft bone into her foot, and torn pelvic-floor muscles to become an Olympian and then a top television commentator (see pages 34–35)
- Fiona Ford, a triathlete badly injured in a collision with a vehicle, subsequently reached the podium at the Ironman World Championships in Kona (she's on pages 54–55).

How are these athletes able to rise again after injuries that might cause others to crumble? The key is what happens when athletes reach critical, difficult moments in their injury process, from the first symptom onward. For some, each one becomes an opportunity to rebound.

In physics, a "rebound" occurs after a collision. Say you drop a red bouncy ball from the top of a gym riser. First, the ball speeds toward the floor; at the moment of impact, all its energy is still moving downward. Then, after the ball hits the ground, there is a transfer of that energy—a momentum shift. The ball changes direction and accelerates back upward.

As a healthy athlete, you might feel like you're moving along in one direction just fine, training and competing in your sport. Then—blammo! You get injured, and it feels like you've hit the floor. Your injury represents a major collision point, and then you might face a few more bumps, such as surgeries, new pains, and fears of re-injury. After each impact, where does your energy go?

During the injury and recovery process, you'll encounter many tough moments. Your setbacks can seem too enormous to overcome; you might lack the support you need to make progress. In those times of struggle, your energy is moving downward. You may sink a bit deeper into doubt, fear, and depression. You can feel as if you're deflating with a splat.

But in every challenging set of circumstances, there are ways—even small ones—to regain control and take action. You might test out a positive mantra, reframe a goal, ask specifically for a type of support you need, or even just pause for a moment before reacting to a piece of bad news. In that moment, you begin to transfer energy from the fall to the bounce—increasing your odds of rising again, and this time even higher.

These responses seem to come almost naturally to certain athletes. Indeed, studies have linked personality traits that scientists have long perceived as relatively fixed to a swifter and more complete recovery from injury. For instance, athletes who score high on a trait called hardiness—a personality type characterized by resilience under stress—appear more likely to experience personal growth after getting hurt.

But if mindset were entirely predetermined by genetics or even by how your parents raised you, Carrie and other mental training coaches and sport psychology pros wouldn't have much of a career. Fortunately, that's not the case, and research has begun to bear out what clinicians like her have long known to be true: **you can work on your mental skills to improve your injury experience**.

A review of the literature by Australian scientists, published in the *British Journal of Sports Medicine*, found that athletes with positive psychological responses to their injury were more likely to return to their sport. Other research has shown that deliberate focus on practices like goal-setting, imagery, and positive self-talk can affect how well, and how swiftly, athletes recover.

In one recent study of a diverse group of athletes from the United States, the United Kingdom, and Finland, almost three-fourths of those who reported using mental skills after their injury said that doing so helped them recover more quickly. But not everyone knows about these skills—in that same study, of more than 1,200 athletes surveyed, only one-fourth had experience applying these psychological techniques.

Fortunately, you'll soon see how mental skills empower you to shift your momentum from the downward plunge and impact of injury to the upward trajectory of your recovery. Instead of crumpling or smashing, you can bounce back stronger. In other words: you can REBOUND.

Through Carrie's work as a clinician and Cindy's as a journalist, as well as through our personal experience with injuries, we've come to understand a few key points:

- Injuries suck, and the impact is mental as much as it is physical.
- Focusing on mental fitness as well as physical rehab is critical to a successful recovery.
- Few injured athletes receive psychological support as they navigate the process.
- Those with superior mental skills often come back mentally and physically stronger—within their sport and beyond it—achieving remarkable recovery.

Every day in her work, Carrie demystifies the machinations of injured athletes' minds. Through the types of mental skills and drills she teaches and prescribes, athletes optimize their mental performance just as they would their physical abilities and techniques. Now, with this book, we're sharing the same strategies that have helped her counsel hundreds of athletes back from the brink and through the rebound, toward a remarkable recovery. We'll also highlight bounce points in many of the athletes' stories we share—places where they hit a bump, then used mental skills to come back stronger.

Injury is difficult, but not hopeless. To rebound you must:

- Understand that injury is mental *and* physical
- Believe that your mindset affects your recovery
- Embrace your power to positively influence your trajectory.

You may not bounce back in exactly the same direction, or in the direction you'd planned. But you *can* bounce back. Ultimately, your life may be better because of it.

Let's explore how a few real-life athletes used mental skills to REBOUND.

The power of psychology

Injury led to Allie Kieffer's first retirement from running. She ran well at Wake Forest University, but repeatedly developed stress fractures in her foot. After graduation, she qualified for the Olympic Trials in the 10,000 meters, but a stress fracture in her tibia prevented her from competing. Soon afterward, she left Boulder, Colorado, the endurance sports mecca, to go back home to New York and a full-time job outside of athletics.

Still, she wasn't quite done with the sport. She began training again—first on her own, then through a Nike program for promising athletes. That boost led to a breakthrough 2:29:39 in the TCS New York City Marathon in 2017—a 26-minute personal best that was good enough for fifth place overall, and second-fastest American, winner Shalane Flanagan being the fastest.

Kieffer returned to running full-time, but did nearly everything differently from before. She minimized stress in her life by dropping destructive relationships and by using tools such as a meal delivery service. (You can formulate your own list of calming strategies using the Stress Busters drill on page 115.) She chose sponsors, including Oiselle, who paid less upfront but offered greater security, should she encounter a setback.

And when she did hit a bump—another stress fracture, in the spring of 2018—she leveraged her resources to cope. She sought help from trusted advisors affiliated with her sponsors, and also shared the news and her struggles on social media. "I've been really open a lot about the bad—but then trying to turn it into a positive too," she said. "It's therapeutic. Maybe I can't fix my bones by talking about it, but I can definitely fix my emotional side." (You can get in touch with your injury-related feelings using the Emotion Decoder on pages 28–29.)

By the summer of 2018, she was racing again—and well. She set personal bests in the 5K in June and the 15K in July, won silver at the 20K National Championships in September, and returned to the New York Marathon in 2018. There, she shaved another minute-plus off her time, running a 2:28:12 and finishing seventh.

Most remarkably, she's even come to feel fortunate for having had her injuries, and particularly for their timing. "I'm lucky it happened now," she said, as it means she can adjust the underlying flaws in her biomechanics in time to attempt to qualify for the Tokyo Olympics in 2020. The path might not be smooth, she knows—in March 2019, she developed more stress fractures in her foot. But she continues to take each injury as an opportunity to re-evaluate her commitment to the sport and an opportunity to return even stronger. In an Instagram post announcing one setback, she quoted Ryan Holiday's book *The Obstacle is the Way*: "These obstacles are actually opportunities to test ourselves, to try new things, and ultimately, to triumph." (Begin to understand how to view your own setbacks as assets by using the Obstacles to Opportunities drill on pages 46–47.)

Dr. Greg Wells was fifteen and en route to the Canadian Olympic Trials in swimming when he attended a training camp in Florida. While he was bodysurfing with his teammates in the ocean, he hit his head and broke his neck in multiple places. After surgery, doctors told him he would never swim again. Wells had other ideas: "From that instant, every single thing was about getting back in the water," he told us. After all, the Trials were just a little over a year away.

Wells went to physiotherapy three to four times a week to strengthen his muscles. Just as important, he recalled, was keeping his mind engaged and staying connected to his teammates so that they could continue to fuel his motivation and mood. (Construct your own support system with the Build Your Team drill on page 133.) Even when all he could do was sit on deck and watch, he still went to practice.

All his hard work paid off: Wells did, in fact, swim in the Olympic Trials in 1992, where he finished tenth. He eventually qualified for the Canada Games, then swam at the University of Calgary. And he even wound up at the Olympics eventually—on the media staff for TSN, a Canadian sports network, a gig that eventually led to a role commentating on the 2010 and 2012 Games.

Now, as an exercise physiologist, broadcaster, and author of such books as *Superbodies: Peak Performance Secrets from the World's Best Athletes*, Wells has seen what it takes for elite athletes to make remarkable recoveries, emerging from injury to the highest echelons of their sport. "If you have a negative mindset, you have essentially no chance of coming back. The positive mindset is the foundation," he said.

- - -

As a freshman on the Sonoma State University basketball team, Molly Donovan had several tears in the labrum of her shoulder repaired. The lifelong athlete had never before had to sit out of competition for an injury, and she found the experience emotionally devastating.

During her second year, she tore her shoulder again, then her anterior cruciate ligament (ACL) and meniscus. Staring down yet another lengthy recovery, this time Donovan chose a different reaction. She found her way to a support group Carrie led on campus, where she felt an immediate kinship with other sidelined athletes. She learned to breathe, relax, and visualize herself succeeding instead of dwelling on her pain and failure. "Injury is about 90% mental. So if you just think about it constantly hurting, it's going to constantly hurt. But if you think about strengthening, then you're going to feel stronger." (Practice this mindset shift with the Feel and Focus drill on page 89.)

Donovan was hurt several more times. During her senior year, she sprained her ankle, a setback that should have scuttled her season. But using her mental skills, she rehabbed aggressively and returned to the court for her final game. "That night, more than anything, I was just proud," she said. She thought back on all she'd overcome and the way she'd mentored other, younger athletes, and realized she could view her athletic career as a success—even if she hadn't racked up as many points or minutes of court time as she'd once hoped.

Post-graduation, mental skills like visualization, goal-setting, and motivation continue to pay off for Donovan. Using imagery, she aced ten interviews to land her first corporate job. (Learn how to craft your own winning imagery script on pages 157–158.) She still sticks notes with motivating quotes in her notebooks and planners, messages that keep her focused and positive. (Try a similar drill, Random Reminders, on pages 91–92.) "Focusing my energy on what I could do to help people versus *woe is me* really strengthened my mindset," she said. "My injuries definitely changed me, but changed me in a good way."

THE FIFTEEN ESSENTIAL MENTAL SKILLS FOR INJURY RECOVERY

Through research, Carrie's clinical experience, and interviews with athletes from Olympians and pro football players to yogis and age-group triathletes, we've identified fifteen mental skills that aid in injury recovery. That might sound overwhelming at first, but think of it this way—that's fifteen different ways you can take control of your injury process and steer it in a healthy, positive direction, to rebound instead of landing flat.

The stories, explanations, and exercises in this book will help you understand and develop these skills. Some are easier to master than others; over time, they build on each other, with rookie skills developing first, then the more advanced levels. One good way to start your mental rehab is to read over this list and identify the skills you suspect are your strengths and those where you know you'll want to do some additional work. You'll find plenty of ways to address each one in the chapters and the forty-nine mental drills that follow.

LEVEL 1 SKILLS—ROOKIE

Confidence	Belief and trust in your ability to accomplish your goals
Focus	Capacity to direct or redirect your energy and attention to what's relevant and constructive
Goal-Setting	Ability to define what you want to accomplish and create a plan to achieve that target
Motivation	Drive and desire to put in the work and push toward your goals and aspirations
Stress Management	Proficiency at using coping skills and strategies to eliminate stressors when you can and to regulate the stress response when you can't

LEVEL 2 SKILLS—ALL-STAR

Attitude	Positive approach and mindset to facing adversity, challenges, and setbacks
Communication	Competence at clearly expressing your opinions and ideas—and ability to hear and understand others' perspectives
Emotional Intelligence	Ability to recognize emotions, discern their origins, and understand how they affect behavior
Self-Awareness	Conscious knowledge about how you operate, including how you think, feel, and react
Visualization	Skillfulness at creating and recreating vivid, controllable images in your mind

LEVEL 3 SKILLS—HALL OF FAME

Discipline	Persistence in pursuit of longer-term goals and deeper values
Generosity	Willingness to extend grace toward yourself and others
Mindfulness	Adeptness at keeping your consciousness in the present moment—or at bringing it back there—and acting as an objective observer of your own experience
Psychological Flexibility	Willingness and ability to adapt to changing circumstances by shifting your reactions, behaviors, and perspective
Resilience	Power to bounce back from hardship or adversity and thrive despite setbacks

Don't worry if some of these sound complex, confusing, or out of your reach. Remember back to the athlete you were when you first started in your sport, and how much better you became with training. Mental skills work much the same way. For each one, you start where you are and gradually hone your technique. Over time, each drill and skill will come that much more easily.

HOW TO USE THIS BOOK

Within these pages, you'll find a wealth of information, including:

◆ Narratives describing athletes' journeys through injury—including highlighted bounce points where they used mental skills (those sections marked "Did you catch the rebound?")
◆ Scientific explanations of the psychological effects of injuries and the mental skills that address them
◆ Key points to take away from each chapter
◆ Specific mental drills you can incorporate throughout your recovery to build those skills.

You might want to start by reading through the whole thing, noting what sounds most like it applies to you and flagging it to study and try later. Every athlete's journey through injury is unique, but understanding the scope of what might occur can offer you a valuable perspective on what to expect and how to prepare, as well as the hope that you'll be able to handle it.

If you're more of a facts-only type, or if reading narratives about others' injuries is painful or stressful for you, you can easily skip over the athletes' stories. You can also start by looking through the "Just the Facts" lists at the end of each chapter for the critical messages, and then flip back through the chapters that pertain most to where you are right now.

From there, you can use the Mental Skills and Drills sections to start building your very own mental rehab plan. Some of the exercises are designed to be done once to guide you through a specific point in time; with others, you'll benefit from regular repetition, just like a physical drill you'd do during practice. Others, as you'll read in the instructions, can stay in your back pocket as ways to help you address particularly challenging situations.

Not every drill will work for every athlete, but we'd encourage you to try as many as possible. You might be surprised by the powerful reaction you have to something you thought sounded a little out there or cheesy. (You can also download a workbook from www.injuredathletesclub.com that will give you a little space to write in.)

We also hope you'll keep this book on the shelf for years to come, long after your injury has become a distant memory. As we noted, a lot of these drills benefit from repeated use, and their value can increase or change at different points in your recovery process. Many serve as potent performance enhancers once you're back to training and competing. And as you'll see in many of the athletes' stories (and learn more about in Chapter 9), you can use them to tackle just about any obstacle you'll face in life. Indeed, nearly every athlete we talked with found that, in some way, they walked away from their experience a better, stronger person, both within their sport and outside of it.

JOIN THE CLUB

Research tells us that one of the most serious psychological consequences of injury is isolation. Coaches (and teammates) can often exacerbate this sensation by acting in a dismissive way: "You're injured? Well, go take care of that and we'll see you when you get better. Hurry up because we need you, but don't come back until you can perform." Sometimes you even "dismiss" yourself, because it's painful to be with people who remind you of what you can't do.

This intense loneliness can leave you feeling as if you're the only injured athlete in the world. But of course, many people out there have been in your shoes—the same shoes you have to hang up for a while until you're back on your feet. Injury also leaves you feeling helpless, consumed by thoughts of all of the things you can't do and are missing out on.

We are here to tell you: You're not alone and you're not helpless. There are many things you can do to help your recovery and to maintain your athletic mindset, even if you lack the support you might wish to receive from the people around you.

And you've already done the first of them: Picking up this book. The information, the athletes' stories, the mental skills, and the mental drills you'll find here will help you address the psychological impact of being injured so you can remain positive and resilient as you rebound.

The best athletes in the world have come to see that they can transform what seems like bad luck into good fortune, and with time and attention, you can too. But don't just take it from us.

The opportunity of injury

Elite marathoner Shalane Flanagan had to drop out of the Boston Marathon in the spring of 2017 with a sacral stress fracture. The ten weeks she took off from running restored her, body and mind. She went on to win the TCS New York City Marathon that fall—the first American to do so since 1977. "Sometimes we don't realize the moment when we feel like dreams are taken away that actually there's some delayed gratification down the road," she said post-race. "I think it was a blessing that I got injured this past winter, and I came here full of energy and motivation and desire to put on the best performance of my life."

NFL star Drew Brees tore his labrum and sustained additional rotator cuff damage in the last game of the 2005 season; his surgically repaired arm would become a liability in future contract negotiations. But in 2006, he signed with the New Orleans Saints. Within a few years he led the team, representing a town, still rebuilding after Hurricane Katrina, to an emotionally significant Superbowl victory. Now, he is recognized as one of the league's greatest quarterbacks. "Many people would define 'the good life' as one that's free of pain and hardship and heartache," he wrote in his 2011 book, *Coming Back Stronger: Unleashing the Hidden Power of Adversity*. But as the title suggests, his injuries have taught him otherwise. "The difficulties life throws at you can be a doorway to something better—something you hadn't even dreamed was possible."

Olympic gold medalist Lindsey Vonn retired in 2019 with a list of injuries that ranged from a cut thumb on a champagne bottle to a crash that required an airlift off the mountain during the Turin Olympics in 2006 (she competed forty-eight hours later), with plenty of broken bones and torn ligaments in between. But in her mind, she might not have had all her successes—and a career that's left her widely regarded as the best skier in history—without them. "Injuries make me appreciate what I do so much more ... every time I've been injured it's made me that much more hungry to get back and be on the mountain again," she's said. "I think every setback is an opportunity to be stronger and a better athlete and also a better person."

CHAPTER 1

INJURIES SUCK

"There's this physical piece of being injured, not being able to push your body, that is one athletes struggle with a lot. But it also brings these emotional pieces we can literally run away from when we're feeling healthy. When we have to slow down, they're more in the forefront, and just as important as your physical limitations."
—*Hillary Allen, professional mountain runner*

There's no doubt about it: getting hurt sucks. It's painful, of course, and physically limiting. But injury involves far more than muscles and bones, tendons and ligaments—it's a full-body physical, mental, and emotional experience. As the days, weeks, and months ahead of you unfold, you might alternate between periods of disappointment, hope, grief, numbness, frustration, and even relief. Acknowledging and allowing yourself to sit with those emotions—and have your feelings heard by others—is an essential first step in moving forward.

Rising again

Hillary Allen had spent three nights in a hospital bed in Norway before she came to a startling realization: The athlete everyone kept talking about—the one who'd tumbled off a mountain during the Hamperokken Skyrace 50K—was her. "It was almost like I was out of my body, on painkillers," she told us in an interview months later. When reality hit her, she said, "I remember thinking, 'Oh crap, this is going to be a long recovery.'"

Somewhere between two checkpoints, at 21.5 and 26.5 kilometers, the runner, surefooted enough to earn the nickname "Hillygoat," took a wrong step off a treacherous stretch on the Hamperokken Ridge.

The 150-foot fall happened so fast Allen didn't even have time to brace herself. She fractured her wrists, two ribs, and two vertebrae in her lumbar spine; sprained her left ankle; and tore a ligament in her right foot, an injury that required two screws to set and heal properly. Hundreds of stitches held her body together.

Allen posted an Instagram video from that Norwegian hospital bed on August 8, 2017, right around the time she'd begun to wrap her head around her new reality. Tubes extend from her head and neck; her arm appears to be encased in what looks like a metal cage.

She was right about her recovery—it was long and difficult. She couldn't walk for two months. With two broken wrists, she also couldn't use crutches, so she procured a red scooter to get around on (to the front, she affixed a Wonder Woman figurine). She didn't run again until November, and then, following a second surgery to remove the screws in her feet, she was grounded for a couple months more.

But what challenged Allen even more than the pain and immobility was the psychological battle that came along with it. At times, she found herself feeling isolated, angry, and depressed. She questioned her identity, her very purpose on the planet without the sport she'd come to love. "I felt days waking up in the morning where I just didn't want to keep going, I wanted to give up … like, if this is what life is going to look like for me, I just don't want any part of it," she said.

The depths to which she sank caught Allen off guard. Not only was she normally an optimist, she'd never been *just* a runner. She came to the sport relatively late, after attending college on a tennis scholarship. She earned a master's degree in neuroscience, still teaches science courses at a community college, and maintains a passion for insects and amphibians, among other creatures.

One reason she loved running was the sense of community it gave her. So when she found herself battling demons of grief and depression, she chose not to hide until everything was fine. From that first video, she spoke openly about the difficult emotions to her friends and family, and to her tens of thousands of social media followers.

The raw honesty of the conversation—not to mention the positive pings from those who liked and commented—proved powerfully healing. Fueled by that momentum, Allen implemented other steps to tend to her emotional well-being. Each day included not only mobility exercises and strength work, but also something solely meant to bring joy—wearing her favorite shirt, getting a cup of coffee from her local shop, sleeping an extra hour.

In June 2018, ten months after her accident, Allen raced again, in the Broken Arrow Skyrace in Squaw Valley, California. She took second place in the VK, a 5-kilometer race with 3,100 feet of vertical gain, and sixth place in the 52K. A week later, she raced again, at the Cortina Trail 48K in the Dolomite Mountains in Italy—and won.

Stepping onto the podium, she's brought with her an entirely new appreciation of how to balance her life, how to thrive around and outside running in addition to within it. They were lessons she put to good use when, eighteen months after her tumble, she fell again and broke her fibula. "Of course, I'm angry and disappointed and the transition to recovery is difficult—and it's certainly not automatic— but I am happy to do it," she wrote at the time. "I know I'll learn something from it—I'm positive of that. It's an opportunity for growth, to learn—that's progress."

Did you catch the rebound? Allen bounced when she decided to be open and transparent about her injury and the difficult emotions that came with it instead of hiding it. She bounced again when she crafted a specific plan for her mental recovery, including building in moments of joy and forgiving herself for days that didn't go perfectly.

Hurt.

Broken.

Damaged.

Sidelined.

Out. Done. Finished.

Whatever words you choose to use, the facts remain the same: You're injured. The minute you crash and fall, see the MRI film, or hear the words from your doctor, trainer, or coach, your heart sinks. The anguish, the disappointment, the despair … no athlete wants to think about it, let alone go through it.

This chapter will explain why you cannot deny the emotional part of the experience any more than you can wish away a fracture or a sprain. We'll show you how to access your emotions, move through them, and then direct your momentum toward the next phase of your rebound.

THE SHOCK OF THE FALL

If you're fortunate enough to call yourself an athlete—especially one who pushes hard to achieve your full potential—you'll likely deal with injury. Yet despite its near ubiquity, injury is one of the more challenging and isolating experiences you will face as an athlete.

Why is this? Although athletes know the possibility of injury comes with the territory, most don't think about it until they actually get hurt. You don't show up to practice each day wondering when your time will come, whether today will be the day you get your first (or next) sprain, tear, or break. You may intuitively understand that when you push your body to the limit, sometimes you find out what that limit is. Day to day, though, most of your attention is dedicated to performing at your best, not to contemplating your odds of a setback.

So when it finally happens to you, injury can come as a profound shock. And the consequences aren't just physical (just ask any athlete who's been through the experience). You've crossed the line from having that athletic mindset of feeling indestructible to deeply and immediately realizing your vulnerability—and that's only the first of many blows to your psyche that injury represents.

THE INJURY ROLLER COASTER

From the moment your injury occurs to the day you play your first game again, or enter your first competition—as well as beyond that day—you will have experienced hundreds, if not thousands, of shifts in your emotional state.

You might feel angry, helpless, disappointed, sad, frustrated, guilty, confused, resilient, strong, excited, hopeful—and you might feel all those in the same day!

Some of these emotions can be confusing or difficult to accept or express. When you're used to training for strength or speed, you might cringe at the thought of weakness or helplessness. Moments when you expressed anger may embarrass you later on, when you're calmer. And though it's obvious that injury is a serious setback in an athlete's life, you might contemplate those who "have it worse" and then feel guilty about your sadness or frustration. For all these reasons, and more, athletes often fight their emotions, deny them, or stuff them deep down inside.

While strategies like reframing and positive self-talk are useful—and we'll get to them later in the book—they tend not to work if you don't first acknowledge your emotions (even the not-so-positive ones). In fact, research—as well as experience—tells us that admitting, rather than burying, your emotions is what enables you to work through them.

For example, British researchers recently asked thirty injured athletes to either talk about their feelings, write about them, or merely to keep a time log of their days for a month. They then interviewed the athletes to assess something called sport-injury-related growth—essentially, the positive changes that come from injury, such as more mental toughness, greater physical strength, better relationships, and increased empathy. After just four weekly twenty-minute sessions, the athletes who had disclosed their emotions (by either talking or writing about them) showed more signs of growing and learning from their recovery, according to the results published in the *Journal of Applied Sport Psychology*. (There's a similar journaling exercise you might want to try a bit later in your injury journey, in Chapter 4, on pages 92–93.)

THE STAGES OF (INJURY-RELATED) GRIEF

Another common emotion that may surprise you in your recovery process is a sense of loss, as if a part of you is suddenly gone. Decades ago, Swiss-born psychiatrist Dr. Elisabeth Kübler-Ross began chronicling the conversations she had with patients upon their realization that they were terminally ill. Although each individual's life, and story, were unique, she identified some common patterns to the way they processed their imminent passing. In 1969, she wrote a groundbreaking book about her work, *On Death and Dying*.

Years later, as sport psychology researchers began delving deeper into the emotional impact of injury, they found striking similarities between sidelined athletes and what Dr. Kübler-Ross had observed among the dying. In both cases, people were processing loss; they were grieving.

The parallel strikes some as a bit dramatic—but you, the injured athlete, know otherwise. When you dedicate so many hours to training and competing, perhaps even banking your livelihood on your athletic performance, your sport becomes central to who you are. This athletic identity extends far beyond the edges of the field or the walls of the locker room, permeating everything you do as a person. Your entire experience of the world—the way you make sense of what's going on around you—hinges on the movement of your body. Having some of your physical capabilities stripped away, even temporarily, leaves a gaping hole.

Researchers have shown that the athletes who take injury the hardest have the highest degree of athletic identity, defining, and explaining, themselves primarily through the lens of their sport. If that strikes a chord with you, see if you can recognize your experience through the five stages of grief: denial, anger, bargaining, depression, acceptance:

DENIAL

Denial usually occurs at the onset of your injury. You're in shock—and that can lead to disbelief. You may even ignore the signals your body is sending and refrain from telling anyone else about them.

Denial differs depending on the type of injury. For acute injuries—those that strike suddenly and are immediately apparent, such as severe tears or serious crashes—you may think:

"No, no, no, no, no."

"This can't be happening."

"Why now? Why is this happening to me?"

For overuse injuries that develop more slowly, or even for acute injuries that don't seem that serious at first, your thoughts may look more like:

"It's OK. Maybe it's not that bad."

"I'll just go home and ice it. It'll probably be fine in a couple of days."

"I'm not going to even bother my coach or trainer with this one. I'm sure it will go away."

Denial is your brain's way of protecting you from emotions you feel unable to handle. Many athletes end up playing through injuries because of this powerful defense mechanism, thereby worsening them and delaying recovery.

ANGER

Now, you're mad. You may blame yourself, or rage at anyone—or anything—you believe played a role in your injury. You're frustrated with your limited mobility, incensed at the idea that you might have to ask people for help. When you see other—uninjured—athletes, you can't help but fume. Often, your greatest rage is directed toward the situation in general—you're furious and resentful that this has happened to you.

BARGAINING

You've let go of some of your anger, and you're not in complete denial—but still, in this stage, you're not quite ready to fully accept your injured status. So, you try to strike a deal, such as:

"I'll take two days off, then pick back up where I left off."

"Maybe it's a little worse than I thought, but I will definitely be back in three weeks before the championship game."

You're attempting to negotiate because you aren't yet ready to accept things as they are. However, you might also begin to think about things you could've done differently that might have prevented the injury.

DEPRESSION

At this stage, the reality of the injury hits you—the truth sinks in. You can't deny or explain away your injury, and the consequences seem devastating and overwhelming. At times, all you can think about is the fact that you can't train or compete; your motivation to work on rehab or recovery may feel nonexistent.

Cut off from your teammates and many of your normal social outlets, you're also likely to feel lost and alone. Compared with non-injured athletes, you're at a higher risk of mood disorders like depression and anxiety; in fact, depression is one of the most common emotional states injured athletes experience. (Sometimes, it's too much to handle on your own. See the box on page 25 for signs that you need help from a mental-health professional.)

When you reach the stage of depression, you've brought yourself into the present moment, as uncomfortable as it may be. You realize that the original goals you had and the path you envisioned are no longer attainable. Though you might feel you've bottomed out, in truth, you're closer to acceptance than you have been at any previous stage. **Allowing yourself to really feel the loss of your goals and your athletic ability is often an essential step in turning the corner toward active recovery.**

ACCEPTANCE

The final stage is acceptance. Negative emotions subside, or at least fade into the background, as you accept your injury and focus on moving forward. You understand that, for the time being, this is your new normal.

Note that acceptance is different from resignation. When you *resign* yourself to the fact that you're injured, you can feel like you're giving up or giving in, that you're stagnant. But when you *accept* that you're injured, you're making an active choice. You may still be disappointed, but you're also ready to do what you need to do to move through this phase of your recovery.

The five stages are listed in linear order, but you might not move through them in that order. Your journey may take you back and forth between stages, or you might skip a stage altogether. However, simply recognizing the possibility that you are grieving a loss can help provide you with some context for your emotional reactions to the experience. You're not crazy just because you've had moments of denial and bargaining. Feeling depressed for a while doesn't mean you will always feel that way. Anger is completely understandable, but it doesn't have to consume you. These are normal reactions to what you're going through as you ponder, "Who am I if I'm not an athlete?" Recognizing them as such immediately begins to put them in a larger perspective.

It's also normal if you don't identify with these stages. Although many injured athletes resonate with them, others might not. Everyone reacts and responds to injury differently—and if you're hurt more than once, you might even have a dramatically different experience each time.

Some athletes move relatively neatly through the stages of grief, while others follow a different path to acceptance. Here are two examples of athletes whose trajectories differed.

The many routes to rebound

The first time Michael Neal tore his ACL, he was just seventeen, and recently drafted to the National Hockey League from the Canadian junior leagues. The second time, he was twenty-seven and a veteran forward for the Indy Fuel, a Chicago Blackhawks affiliate. Here's how the stages unfolded for his second injury:

Denial: All these years later, Neal still wore the brace he got from his previous surgery. Over and over, he told himself: "I had a brace on, there's no way anything could happen." The doctor who checked him soon afterward, in the training room, told him it seemed like his hamstring, not his knee; though he suspected otherwise, Neal was tempted to believe him.

Anger: The next day, his trainer texted him, asking if he was coming to the game. Neal thought the question odd, until he arrived at the rink and the trainer invited him into the office, then pointed to the MRI image on the screen. Neal read the words "ruptured ACL." He processed the news calmly, then went to his truck to call his girlfriend. He might have let a swear word or two loose, lost in rage against the other player and above all the situation.

Bargaining: When Neal went to get his MRI, he chatted with the technician a bit about what she saw, hoping she'd reveal a clue. All she'd let slip was that she could see he'd had surgery on his ACL before. "I got excited because I thought, well, if she can see that, she must be able to see my ACL," he said—letting this raise his hopes that the ligament was still intact. Indeed, he almost called his parents to tell them the worst-case scenario was off the table.

Depression: For a while, Neal stayed in his truck, bawling. That night, he hit the town to "blow off some steam," commiserating with some of his teammates.

Acceptance: During a calmer and less emotional talk with his girlfriend later, Neal evaluated his options. He'd been playing better than ever and felt on the verge of a breakthrough season. No, he decided, he wasn't done playing hockey. He'd overcome setbacks before and could do so again. The next day he saw the physical therapist to begin prehab for surgery.

The road ahead involved more low moments—including sitting alone in Indianapolis for hours each day in severe pain post-surgery—as well as highs, like returning to the ice. Neal came back to competition after seven months, was named the team captain, and despite having missed the first six games, ended the season as the Fuel's top scorer, racking up twenty goals and thirty-two assists.

- - -

Elite marathoner Alia Gray didn't follow such a clear journey through the stages of grief when she developed a sacral stress fracture in 2017. She already knew she was tough; she'd logged up to ninety miles per week on an AlterG anti-gravity treadmill before the 2016 Olympic Trials marathon after suffering a fractured fibula from an ankle roll. In fact, those lonely miles in a non-air-conditioned room likely paid off for her during the race itself, in which dozens of runners dropped out due to high temperatures—Gray placed 10th.

When Gray felt a sharp pain in her back one Wednesday in December 2017, she knew something was very wrong. Gray has an advantage over some other athletes: she's married to Dr. Richard Hansen, a chiropractor and coach of the Roots Running Project in Boulder. She was able to get an MRI two days later, on Friday.

With each beep the magnets made, Gray hoped for the best. "I remember just thinking like, 'Please, please, please, please, please' on every single buzz, like just kind of pleading that it wasn't anything big," she told us in an interview. And when the results came back clean, she was thrilled.

She took a week of rest, but the pain worsened. The next week, she got another MRI; this one showed the break in her bone. "By that point, I was just ready for an answer," she said. "In a way, I would've been upset if it came back normal again. It was so clear that something was off." When she looks back at her journal entries from that time, she notes a yo-yo of emotions—exhaustion from trying to figure out answers (and from a recently diagnosed chronic sinus infection), fear and nervousness about whether she would have the ability to come back from what would be her longest-ever break, relief at the notion of being able to take some rest and read some books, and then guilt about feeling that relief.

Mixed in, though, were periods of peace with what her body was telling her, and a knowledge that she was in the best possible position to move ahead. With that relatively swift move to acceptance, she forged ahead. By mid-April, she was logging easy miles again; in July, she took part in her first race since her injury, the famous Boilermaker 15K in Utica, New York, and placed fourteenth. "Allowing yourself appropriate time to grieve the injury and missed training is super important, but it's also important to be aware enough to not allow that to be your new normal operating control," she said. "Checking in with myself and having others to check in on me helped me find that balance."

YOU MUST BE THIS TALL TO BOARD

In addition to outlining patterns, like the stages of grief, that many injured athletes have in common, researchers are also working to understand what makes them all different from each other. Why does injury take some only on the equivalent of a kiddie coaster with just a few dips and rises, while others have an experience akin to a terrifying gut-clencher (with a busted safety belt thrown in)?

Here's what they've noticed: As you contemplate your injury, you size up the situation and determine whether or not you have what it takes to face it. This assessment—sometimes conscious, sometimes not—plays a key role in both how you feel about your injury and what you do about it. When this calculation happens below the level of awareness, you risk basing it on fears and assumptions as opposed to facts and truths. So, let's shine a little light on what your brain's going through at this point.

Of course, the type of ride you're boarding makes a difference to how you cope—that is, the basic characteristics of your athletic career, the injury that's interrupted it, and the external resources you have to handle what you're going through. Researchers call these situational factors, and they include:

◆ the type, and the severity, of the injury
◆ the timing of the injury
◆ your level of competition
◆ your access to rehabilitation resources
◆ your support system
◆ the nature of your interactions with your healthcare team
◆ whether your injury is invisible (which can lead you to worry about others questioning whether you really are injured) or visible (which provides a constant reminder of the things you can't do).

But some of your inherent skills and characteristics—things specific to you, the athlete stepping onto this often unpredictable ride—also play a role. These are personal factors, and they include:

◆ your history with injury
◆ the coping skills you have
◆ your athletic identity
◆ your history with stressors
◆ your pain tolerance.

Consider two athletes with very different histories: one has had previous experience of successfully returning from injury, had a short-term injury at the beginning of the season, and has stellar coping skills and a strong support system, including a top-notch doctor and trainer or therapist. The other has never faced an injury, is near the end of a collegiate season (which means they are possibly also near the end of their career), has limited resources and few supportive friends and family, and has a doctor who isn't knowledgeable about treating athletes and a physical therapist who lacks empathy. You can easily see how differently they'd react to the experience of injury.

As with so many other elements of the injury process, simply being aware of these dynamics can dramatically alter your experience of them. But by using the types of skills described in this book, you can go beyond merely understanding your response to injury to actually being able to change that response.

Of course, there are some situational and personal factors you can't change. As any kid who's stood on tippy-toes trying to gain the necessary extra inches to finally get to ride Space Mountain can tell you, the quest to defy physiology doesn't always pan out. You don't always have the freedom or resources to switch your medical team (though we have some ideas for how to handle that on page 130). But many of these factors *are* within your power to influence—such as your coping skills (see pages 101–103), your support system (see page 133), the way you handle fear of re-injury (see pages 171–173), even your pain tolerance (that info's on pages 105–107). What's more, although you can't alter something like your injury history or the timing of your injury, there's a lot you can do to change your reaction to obstacles in ways that benefit your recovery and, ultimately, your well-being.

WARNING: CURVES AHEAD

In addition to scouring the research, we've interviewed more than fifty injured athletes for this book. One of the findings that rings true—across both scientific studies and athletes' experiences—is that a few key points in the process are far more likely than others to produce emotional difficulties. But for reasons we'll delve into in Chapter 2, our brains are hardwired to prefer knowledge to uncertainty, and that means a glimpse of the track ahead, even of the topsy-turvy parts, helps prepare you to navigate it.

So be warned—you're more likely to experience negative emotions when the following apply:

◆ When your injury first occurs (regardless of its severity)
◆ When you experience setbacks during rehabilitation
◆ If you hit a plateau or feel like you're moving backward
◆ When you are cleared to return to full training and competition.

While attention to your psychological recovery is important at every stage of your injury journey, it may be even more critical at those times.

Important note: If your injury involves a concussion, your emotional journey may be different. Concussion is linked to anxiety and depression, and can change the way you mentally process your injury, as well as meaning that you will require rest from any cognitively challenging activities, including mental drills. Turn to Chapter 9 for a little more information about this, and if you have been concussed, be sure to check in with your medical team about when and how it's appropriate to start incorporating mental drills into your rehab.

DEPRESSION AND ANXIETY: WATCH FOR THESE WARNING SIGNS

Depression and anxiety are common among injured athletes, and sometimes become so severe as to interfere with every other aspect of their lives as well. If you find that coping with your injury leaves you feeling so overwhelmed that you can't even imagine a way out, or if you are experiencing the following warning signs, consider seeking help from a mental-health professional:

◆ Withdrawal from social contact
◆ Changes in sleeping and eating habits
◆ Decreased interest in other activities
◆ Problems concentrating, focusing, or remembering
◆ Deliberate self-harm
◆ Irritability
◆ Drug and alcohol abuse
◆ Thinking about death, dying, or going away. If you find yourself contemplating suicide, call the National Suicide Prevention Lifeline at 1-800-273-8255, or chat live, online, 24/7 at suicidepreventionlifeline.org in the United States. U.K. residents, call the Samaritans on 116 123.

GET READY TO REBOUND

What's the measure of successful recovery from an athletic injury? In most cases, it's a successful return to your prior level of training and competition. If that's what you want—to return to your previous sport—we want that for you, too. But we know it isn't always possible—and even if it is, we also want more than that.

We want you to contemplate the fact that you might be able to do more—to rebound feeling amazed by your mental toughness, proud of your strength and perseverance, and perhaps even grateful for your challenges. If you choose, you can use this as an opportunity to build powerful mental skills that not only boost resilience as you recover, but allow you to thrive once you're past it. In short—like so many athletes in this book have done—we want you to emerge from this experience feeling like you are a better and stronger person for it.

Getting there involves accepting that you are injured, taking personal responsibility for your recovery, and believing in your ability to not only get through this difficult time, but to continue to rise beyond it. If you're just at the beginning of your injury journey, that may seem like an incredibly tall order. Fortunately, this book is full of inspirational stories, clear but accurate scientific explanations, and mental drills that enable you to recover mentally as you recover physically. Most of the time athletes focus purely on the physical aspects of recovery and hope the mental side catches up. If you take anything away from this book, we hope it's this: You don't have to leave that catch-up to chance. You can do this, let's get to work.

No longer an underdog

Brandon Copeland always considered himself the underdog. Sure, he had football in his blood—his grandfather had played for eleven years for the Baltimore Colts—and a natural talent had been apparent ever since his mom put aside her fears of him getting hurt and let him onto the field in fourth grade. But he didn't even make junior varsity his first year of high school. Instead of a powerhouse college, he went to the University of Pennsylvania, where he understood he'd have to work harder to earn a spot in the NFL.

And he did, despite sustaining his first major injury—a torn meniscus—six weeks before he was due to perform before NFL scouts at his school's Pro Day. When his knee injury occurred, the linebacker told us in an interview that he remembers calling his mom, crying, "This is what I've been working for, and it's potentially all gone." He took a day or two to sulk, then got to work. For three weeks, he didn't run, focusing only on building upper-body strength. "Then I took three weeks of training all day, every day to get back to where I could give myself a chance." He went undrafted, but signed a three-year contract worth $1.5 million with the Baltimore Ravens.

His career wasn't exactly smooth sailing from there on out. In four years, he was cut five times and signed ten different contracts with three teams. He finally found a place on the Detroit Lions, where he played a key role on special teams and also played both linebacker and defensive end—the multifunctional type of player analysts dubbed a "Swiss Army knife." He began to feel his star rise, and that he was finally getting the respect he'd known he deserved, and with it, the chance to start on a pro team. Then, one Sunday in August during an exhibition game against the Indianapolis Colts, he tore a pec muscle.

He can still hear the sound of his muscle ripping and, with it, his career evaporating. Much as he had done before, he spent a couple of days in a dark room, eating ice cream and watching mindless TV. He knows himself well enough to know he needs these "woe is me" moments, but he also knows he can't linger there too long.

His underdog career path, not to mention his previous injury, had taught Copeland a thing or two. Before he went into surgery the following Thursday, he'd already crafted a comeback playlist on Spotify, which he titled "Rebirth". (Learn how to make your own using the Power Playlists drill on page 182.) That was just one part of the game plan. Music moved him on some days; on others he thought of providing for his family. Sometimes he even flipped back through screenshots of disparaging tweets from trolls. He saves them all, knowing someday he'll flip their negativity into fuel. (Using the Found in Translation drill on page 135 can help you handle difficult interactions with others.)

Though he might not have chosen a torn pec muscle as the path to take him where he's always wanted to be, Copeland ultimately landed there: in New York. After returning to the field, he signed a contract with the Jets in 2018. Following what the *New York Daily News* called a "career year" in 2018—with five sacks and forty-seven tackles—Copeland re-signed in March 2019.

Did you catch the rebound? Copeland bounced when he owned up to his sadness, briefly sulked, then chose to move past it. He bounced again when he planned ahead for all the motivation he'd need to get through rehab.

JUST THE FACTS

- Nearly all athletes—especially those who push hard to achieve their full potential—will likely deal with injury.
- Even if you know injury is an inherent risk, getting hurt can still come as a shock.
- During your injury process, you will experience hundreds, if not thousands, of shifts in your emotional state.
- Some of these emotions can be deep and powerful—you may grieve the loss of your identity.
- Acknowledging, rather than burying, your emotions is what enables you to work through them.
- The injury journey looks different for every athlete depending on both situational and personal factors.
- Your response to injury depends, in part, on whether you feel you have the resources to cope with the challenges ahead of you.
- Using the skills and drills in this book, you can change your response to injury and take active steps to enable you to rebound.

MENTAL SKILLS AND DRILLS

How can you share openly like Hillary Allen, move through the stages of grief like Michael Neal, cultivate a range of uplifting and motivating strategies like Brandon Copeland? These drills allow you to recognize, release, and move through your emotions, succeeding apart from them and not in spite of them.

MENTAL DRILL: EMOTION DECODER

Choose from a master list of emotions—the Emotion Decoder—to accurately label your feelings.

Mental Skills:
Level 1, Rookie: Stress Management
Level 2, All-Star: Emotional Intelligence, Self-Awareness

Emotions are often distinct and nuanced, but we tend to generalize our feelings, clumping them into buckets of "good" and "bad." Labeling the exact feeling you have in a given moment—calling an emotion what it is—can be surprisingly powerful.

Use the Emotion Decoder when you are feeling stuck or upset, or any time you want a little more insight into your state of mind. Sometimes just the act of naming a feeling provides relief, allowing you to move through it and then move on from it. You can also use the Emotion Decoder to help you fill out the first question on your Injury Intake Form (see page 30).

Circle all that you are currently feeling (you'll also find a copy of this list in the workbook, which you can download at www.injuredathletesclub.com):

Accepting	Empowered	Joyful
Adversarial	Envious	Judgmental
Aggressive	Excited	Lonely
Angry	Exhausted	Mad
Annoyed	Fearful	Miserable
Anxious	Foolish	Moody
Ashamed	Frazzled	Panicked
Betrayed	Frightened	Pleased
Bored	Frustrated	Powerful
Brave	Glad	Preoccupied
Calm	Grateful	Proud
Cautious	Grieving	Reactionary
Competitive	Guilty	Rejected
Confident	Happy	Relief
Conflicted	Helpless	Remorseful
Confused	Hopeful	Resentful
Courageous	Hopeless	Responsible
Curious	Hurt	Sad
Defeated	Ignorant	Scared
Depressed	Impulsive	Selfish
Desperate	Indifferent	Sensitive
Determined	Insecure	Shame
Disconnected	Inspired	Shocked
Discouraged	Intolerant	Sorry
Disgusted	Irritated	Tense
Elated	Isolated	Tired
Embarrassed	Jealous	Worried

MENTAL DRILL: INJURY INTAKE FORM

Assess your current psychological state in regard to your injury.

Mental Skill:
Level 2, All-Star: Self-Awareness

Your doctors, trainers, and therapists will gauge where you are physically with your injury, but take the time to get a feel for your psychological status, too. Answering the questions on the Injury Intake Form will help you assess your mental state and start to process your injury experience a bit more deeply, so you can plan where you want to go. Grab a piece of paper (or the workbook, which you can download at www.injuredathletesclub.com), find a quiet spot, and answer the questions below:

1. What are some of the emotions you've experienced with your injury so far?
2. What are some of the specific challenges you've faced in dealing with your injury?
3. What is your biggest fear or concern right now?
4. What do you feel you're doing well in terms of how you're dealing with your injury?
5. Are there any ways you feel you're holding yourself back from progressing with your injury recovery?
6. What personal or situational factors are you experiencing that might be contributing to the stress of being injured?
7. How are you feeling about your medical team?
8. Do you feel there is any additional support you need?

MENTAL DRILL: SIDELINED SWOT

*Catalog the strengths, weaknesses, opportunities, and threats
that will influence your recovery.*

Mental Skills:
Level 1, Rookie: Confidence, Motivation
Level 2, All-Star: Self-Awareness
Level 3, Hall of Fame: Discipline

The SWOT (strengths, weaknesses, opportunities, and threats) analysis was designed for organizations to assess their resources and risks, so that they could make informed decisions when moving forward with their businesses. In this case, you are the organization, and right now your organization is injured. What are your personal strengths, weaknesses, opportunities, and threats as they pertain to your recovery? Start brainstorming and exploring by answering the questions listed in each category (you'll find a blank grid in the workbook). You can use these questions as a starting point, but feel free to keep writing if you want to. Once you have completed your SWOT analysis, take action on your assessment. Use your SWOT analysis to help inform the goals you will be coming up with in Chapter 3.

INJURY SWOT

STRENGTHS	WEAKNESSES
What advantages do you have?	What are you lacking?
What are you feeling confident about?	What could you improve?
What would other people identify as your personal strengths?	What's your biggest frustration?
What personal characteristics are you proud of?	What are you avoiding?
OPPORTUNITIES	THREATS
What are you looking forward to?	What obstacles do you face?
What opportunities do you see?	What fears are holding you back?
What new areas could you be working on?	What is missing?
What positive and healthy habits could you cultivate?	What could further harm you?

MENTAL DRILL: MY CONDOLENCES

Write yourself a sympathy card acknowledging your suffering and loss.

Mental Skills:
Level 2, All-Star: Communication, Emotional Intelligence
Level 3, Hall of Fame: Generosity

If you had a friend going through a rough time, you wouldn't hesitate to send them some snail-mail. Now, extend the same kindness to yourself. Actually go out and buy yourself a card. Write it as if you were addressing a loved one or a best friend, acknowledging the loss you've been feeling.

For example: *"I'm so sorry you're having to face this injury. It really sucks that you have to go through this. I know how important it was to you to do this race. I know you don't want to be facing this and you wish it wasn't happening, but I also know that you are strong, and you can get through this."*

MENTAL DRILL: LAUGH OUT LOUD

Make a list of alternative ways to boost endorphins and seek joy.

Mental Skills:
Level 1, Rookie: Stress Management
Level 2, All-Star: Self-Awareness
Level 3, Hall of Fame: Generosity, Resilience

Injury ranks among the most stressful events you will go through as an athlete; not only are both your body and your mind under duress, but you're often denied the regular endorphin boost that comes with intense physical activity. Proactively seek out these feel-good neurochemicals aids in recovery by countering the stress you're enduring. Take five minutes to create these lists of five (you'll find a space to do so in the workbook):

- What are five things that you know make you smile?
- What are five things most likely to make you laugh out loud?
- What are five activities you enjoy doing that you can do while injured?
- What are five of your favorite television or movie comedies?

Pick at least one to do proactively every day—and add another when you feel like you need to balance out the stress you're feeling.

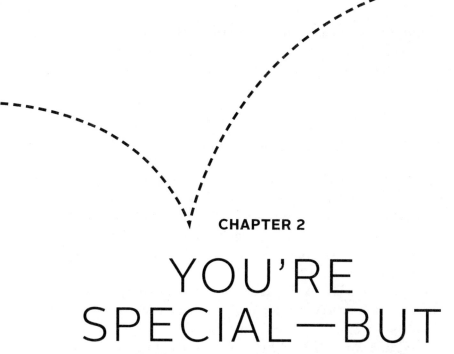

CHAPTER 2

YOU'RE SPECIAL—BUT YOU'RE NOT SPECIAL

"It stinks and there's no way around it when you're injured; it is really tough. But I looked at it as glass half full rather than half empty. And that's how I look at my life—I think, 'How can I become a better runner, better athlete, better person because of these hardships?'"
—*Olympic runner Carrie Tollefson*

Humans' logical brains prefer predictability, a series of events spelled out in black and white. Injuries are unexpected, with shades of gray surrounding their consequences. One day you're at the peak of fitness; the next, you're unable to take a step. Timelines and plans you had painstakingly crafted no longer appear attainable. Instead of a clear-cut competitive schedule, you're left with a series of obstacles and an uncertain timeline. When you think of it this way, there's little wonder it can be so difficult to adjust. But with the right skill set, you can learn to navigate within contradictions and unpredictability—and reap incredibly powerful rewards.

Strength through setbacks

Most injured athletes deal with some level of ambiguity. Runner Carrie Tollefson's first major injury put her entire future in doubt. In 1998, the then-junior at Villanova was aiming for her first NCAA cross-country championship when she went to the doctor with heel pain. An MRI revealed a stress fracture that had already healed—and a tumor measuring more than an inch.

Her doctors couldn't tell whether the growth was benign or cancerous without a biopsy, surgery that might threaten her running career at a key point in her season. So they chose to monitor the situation as she continued to compete. "What I had to do was just to sort of live day by day and know that tomorrow could be taken away," she told us in an interview. She trained harder than ever, and came back to win the cross-country championships again in what she thought might be her last hurrah.

The surgery Tollefson had soon afterward revealed that the tumor wasn't malignant. Her doctors weren't sure what had caused it, but knew that if it didn't come out a wrong step could shatter her heel. So they removed the growth and implanted a bone graft from a donor, which they hoped would encourage new bone to sprout. Tollefson did her part to enhance the process: "I used to talk to that foot all the time—like, 'Come on, grow a new bone, you've got to do this for me,'" she said. (It was her own form of an Injury Mantra—craft one specific to your situation on pages 70–71.)

The treatment required her to take six months off running, but Tollefson returned and went on to thrive, despite having a career that was littered—or as she'd say, "glittered"—with overuse injuries, from stress fractures to torn pelvic floor muscles to a case of plantar fasciitis in her other foot that took eighteen months to heal. After Villanova, she went on to run professionally, and competed in the 1,500 meters in the 2004 Olympic Games in Athens. "I think I became a better athlete because of my injuries. I think I became a tougher person and more perseverant person," she said.

Today, she has a successful career as a commentator, broadcaster, podcaster, and speaker, in addition to overseeing training camps for young athletes. And she's widely known for her compassion—she makes time for personal connections with runners at all levels of the sport, especially those who have overcome adversity themselves.

Did you catch the rebound? Tollefson bounced when she decided to focus on each day instead of on the anxiety of the unknown. She bounced again when she viewed her injuries as opportunities to grow.

Navigating the injury process involves managing these uncertainties, and also learning how to wrap your mind around facts that seem, at first, completely contradictory. For instance: You're special, but you're not special. Obviously you're not the only person who has had to face an athletic injury—many others have endured the frustration, fears, and emotional turmoil that come with being sidelined (so you're *not* special). However, athletes experience and react to their injuries in many different ways—so you *are* special, and you are entitled to your own unique injury experience.

Choosing a positive way to respond to contradictions, doubt, and uncertainty stands as one of the greatest challenges of being hurt. But if you can learn to master it, the resulting shift in perspective can prove immensely powerful.

THE GREAT GRAY ABYSS

If you're like most of the athletes we know, the minute you realize you're hurt, your mind fills with questions. One of the downsides of each of us being unique is that while your medical team and other athletes can inform and inspire you, no one can tell you exactly how—or at what pace—your own recovery will proceed. A major challenge you'll face early on in your injury is how to deal with all of the unknowns:

- How long will my recovery take?
- Will I get my fitness back?
- When will I (or even will I) be able to train and compete again?
- Is there still going to be a spot for me on the team?

◆ Will I be the same athlete I was before my injury?
◆ If I do have to walk away from my sport, who will I then be?

As if the initial unknowns about injury weren't bad enough, sometimes the picture grows even murkier as time passes. Immediately after an injury or surgery, visible signs like crutches and bandages signify your injured status; your primary role may be to rest or closely follow your doctor's orders. That changes as you begin to grow stronger, lose the apparent evidence of your setbacks, and get closer to returning to training and competition. At this point, you're faced with many small decisions about how much to rest and how much to push, and your teammates and training partners may either expect you to perform like you'd never been hurt or pamper you as if you're entirely fragile.

At any point during your injury process, you can get consumed with all of the what-ifs. As well as practical answers to your questions about your recovery, you're also grasping for something deeper—stability, permanence, control. After all, humans like certainty. We're not so cool with the concept of hanging out in the vast unceasing gray.

In her book, *Living Beautifully with Uncertainty and Change*, the American Buddhist nun Pema Chödrön explains the Buddhist concept of groundlessness: the idea that life is uncertain and everything is always changing. We fight against this truth and are constantly grasping to put ground beneath our feet, to have something solid to stand on. Sometimes this means we are willing to endure negative consequences in preference to the angst of not knowing.

Besides just plain making you feel crummy, this trepidation about an uncertain future can affect your recovery in a few different ways:

◆ Quitting prematurely.
◆ Continuing half-heartedly.
◆ Limiting your potential.

QUITTING PREMATURELY

You might decide you would rather walk away from training and competing altogether than live with an unclear outcome or feeling unsure of your next move. The transition away from your sport is a topic we'll cover more in Chapter 8—but in short, while that's a perfectly valid decision to make after an injury (especially a serious one), you don't want to let fear make that decision for you.

For example, Canadian skier Anna Goodman knows she can persevere through injury—she skied in the 2010 Winter Olympics with a torn ACL. Her injury occurred only a month before the Games, meaning she wouldn't have time for surgery and rehab. So she pursued an aggressive strengthening program, put on a big knee brace and, after hitting the slopes a grand total of five times after her injury, came in 19th in slalom. She had surgery, rehabbed, and was back on the snow six months later.

But two subsequent injuries, and their aftermath, led her to retire from the sport at the relatively young age of twenty-six. The last injury, to her hip, proved especially frustrating—she knew something wasn't right, but her coaches and team doctors believed her pain was only muscular. Finally, an MRI she insisted on having revealed a hole in her cartilage that required surgery. She came back from that physically, but mentally, she'd lost her drive.

Goodman's clear that she's not bitter; she had reignited her passion for skiing again after leaving the team, while competing for Westminster College in Salt Lake City, and had been aiming to make the 2014 Olympic team when yet another ACL tear sidelined her again. But now, as a coach and camp director for young female skiers, she emphasizes to them the importance of following their gut, listening to their bodies, and focusing on their long-term goals instead of on short-term obstacles and uncertainties.

CONTINUING HALF-HEARTEDLY

Fear of the unknown can trap you in your existing path, even when your motivations and goals have shifted. This mismatch between your desires and your behaviors can trigger anxiety, depression, or maladaptive coping mechanisms.

This type of scenario occurred for alpine skier Kirsten Cooper. Not long after she made Team USA, she had a terrible crash while training downhill in Chile. As she whizzed down the mountain at around seventy-five miles per hour, she hit a bump, bounced, and landed in a field of rocks, ending up with brain bleeding, six vertebral fractures, five broken ribs, and torn ligaments in her lower back.

After a year-long recovery process, she returned to racing, then stayed on the team for several more years. But inside, she felt her career was over: "I was scared for my life every time I stepped in my skis," she told us. On the one hand, she remembered how hard she'd worked to get where she was, but on the other, she knew her fear and hesitancy increased her risk of crashing again—and if she did, the consequences would be devastating. However, tipping the balance in favor of continuing to race was the fact that her identity was so wrapped up in the sport that the fear of considering another path was nearly unbearable. "It was incredibly painful to be doing what I was doing, but that was so much better than thinking about doing anything else," she said. Looking back, she wishes she could tell her younger self that there was a fulfilling life to be lived on the other side of competing.

LIMITING YOUR POTENTIAL

If you're too quick to search for or accept a firm answer on what you can accomplish after your injury, you might be limiting your options unnecessarily.

Triathlon coach Alistair Robinson, whom we will meet again in Chapter 7, returned to the sport after a severe bike crash that fractured his skull and nine vertebrae. Now he frequently coaches athletes in the post-injury stages, and points out that even the most talented medical team can't decode exactly what's happening in anyone's unique body, in the unique circumstances their injury has imposed upon it. He's seen injured athletes quickly settle for less than complete recovery, accepting when a doctor says, for instance, "You'll always have back pain."

He advises them not to believe such proclamations without question. Though he is the first to admit that not everyone can achieve 100% recovery, he encourages every athlete to consider aiming for it, leaving no stone unturned in their quest for ongoing improvement. "If you look at it as like, I'm going to keep doing everything I can—be it therapy, be it training, be it exploring further medical approaches—you give yourself a chance. If you settle, you give yourself no chance," he told us.

HOW YOUR MIND IS LIKE YOUR MUSCLES

While being human gives us an inherent dislike of dealing with uncertainty, we've also been gifted brains big enough to overcome this deficiency. It isn't easy to do, but the rewards are great. Can you view the unknown as a puzzle to be solved rather than an abyss to be avoided? Instead of feeling like a victim of your injury, could you come to see it as a rite of passage? And then, could you take a step even further, and see it as an opportunity for growth?

Ironically, the first step in this process might be acknowledging just how big an impact your injury has had on you—that it is, in fact, a trauma. For some of you, the term won't resonate, or you might even feel an aversion to it. Portraying injury as a "trauma" might seem like a sign of weakness or as insensitive to people who are experiencing situations you perceive as so much worse.

When we think of trauma, we naturally think of the absolute worst thing someone could be facing. The way we are defining "trauma" here is: *a distressing and challenging experience.* Yes, there are degrees of trauma, and yes, there is someone out there who is likely enduring a more traumatic experience than you. However, that does not diminish what you are going through. Life has dealt you a difficult experience, and acknowledging your negative emotions doesn't mean you're weak, whining, or selfish. It just means you're honest.

Once you can view it in this light, research supports the idea that trauma can inspire emotional and personal growth. You can think of it as similar to muscular growth, a process called hypertrophy. When you apply resistance—when you lift a dumbbell or crank out a round of push-ups—your muscle fibers experience microscopic tears. Your body then goes into action at a cellular level and starts to repair the injury. This process of damage and repair makes your muscles stronger. Your muscles *have to experience trauma in order to grow,* and you can also grow as a person and an athlete in response to trauma.

The idea that you can actually experience positive changes through adversity is also known as "stress-related growth." Are we suggesting that it's awesome that you're currently injured? That's a resounding NO. Are we suggesting that you go out and get injured to experience this stress-related growth? DEFINITELY NOT. What we *are* suggesting is that there may be another way of looking at your injury, a way of perceiving this obstacle as a springboard toward something greater. When you start to make this mindset shift, it can allow you to let go of things that are not in your control and focus on the things you *can* influence or change. It shifts your mindset from trying to grasp for ground underneath you to seeing what ground is still there, and building on it.

FINDING YOUR WAY ACROSS SHIFTING GROUND

So, what makes the difference between resilient athletes who come to view their injuries as opportunities, and those who struggle to cope? Research has pinpointed two important factors: self-compassion and hardiness. While some people naturally possess these attributes to a greater extent than others, anyone can learn to recognize them, nurture them, and more deeply develop them as they navigate their unique—yet universal—injury experience.

SELF-COMPASSION

When you are a compassionate person, you respond with kindness to a person's suffering. You feel what this person is going through. You don't judge this person as they struggle, you show understanding and caring. When you are the recipient of this compassion you feel heard, seen, and understood; you feel supported. When you cultivate *self*-compassion, you turn all of that kindness toward yourself. Cultivating the ability to step outside of yourself and have compassion for this person who is hurting, sad, angry, confused, and struggling—even when that person is staring back at you in the mirror—forms a vital first step in the process toward recovery and growth.

You might need to practice self-compassion when:

- you don't want to see your teammates
- you're angry with people for asking about your injury
- you feel guilty for being upset when you know others are suffering more than you
- you feel jealous of people who *are* able to train and compete
- you feel worried about getting injured again
- you are judging yourself about anything.

When you find yourself caught up in one of these emotions, notice them, then use self-compassion to give yourself a break. You're human and therefore subject to the pains and complicated emotions that afflict every member of our species. Those emotions make being human both beautiful and painful—and beauty and pain are two sides of the same coin. You can't have the ability to experience one without also being willing to endure the other.

Self-compassion offers you a tool to both honor your emotions and objectively see this injury experience for what it is. (We'll give you a specific drill at the end of this chapter—it's called Go FAR—to help you practice it.) When you can step outside of yourself, you can observe yourself without judgment. You don't get overwhelmed by the experience of being injured. You move from "Why is this happening to me? This isn't fair!" to "It sucks that I'm here—and I'd prefer not to be—but I can do this."

HARDINESS

Hardy people are able to cope with stress effectively, and research shows that athletes high in hardiness are more likely than those who are less hardy to experience stress-related growth outcomes as a result of their injuries.

Hardiness comprises three aspects: commitment, control, and challenge.

- ◆ *Commitment* refers to the ability to persevere—to keep putting one foot in front of the other even when faced with difficult times. You stay involved, seeing things through to the end despite any obstacles you may encounter.
- ◆ *Control* refers to the ability to not feel helpless when faced with difficult times. You believe you are capable of influencing the circumstances of your life, understand that certain things are out of your control, and take action to address the things you can influence.
- ◆ *Challenge* is the inclination to view stressors as a normal and ongoing part of life. You know that setbacks are not threats to your safety and security but, rather, challenges and opportunities for deepening your understanding and growth.

Working on self-compassion and hardiness can help you avoid ruminating— that is, staying focused solely on the negative aspects of being injured. The progression of healing, both physically and mentally, is never going to be linear, but with these two critical tools at your disposal, you can keep moving forward in the face of challenges and keep your heart and mind open to possibilities.

The performance mindset

Going into his junior year, University of Pennsylvania football player Joe Holder injured his ankle. He tried to follow the advice of his medical team, but still, his pain lingered and the joint wouldn't heal. Eventually, his coach and teammates came to doubt his toughness and sincerity, and he himself began sinking into depression, partying too hard and slipping, both physically and academically. Holder finally hit a low moment when he forgot to call home on his dad's birthday. That marked a turning point. His father happened to be a holistic physician, and the two worked together to revamp much of Holder's lifestyle, including adopting a plant-based diet and changing his training routine.

Holder also began applying lessons he was learning in a marketing psychology class to his own mindset. He boosted his hardiness by replacing doubts and negative thoughts that had plagued him in the past with productive ones, using techniques like mindfulness training, healing visualizations, and mental contrasting—all of which we'll explore in more depth in Chapter 3 (the Plan B exercise on pages 181–182 is a good example). He practiced self-compassion by imagining how he'd talk to someone else in the same boat—with empathy, not harshness.

Holder's new strategies were put to the test again his senior year, when he broke his leg and was told he'd be out for the year. He gave himself two days to wallow, then launched himself into rehab, both physically and mentally. "I made sure my mindset was super positive. I didn't let anybody keep me down mentally," he said. And it worked. He came back in four weeks to finish out the season.

Today he's a popular, successful coach and personal trainer in New York, working with actors, models, and athletes. He teaches them all the same techniques. "It's just the same thing as when you're practicing football or basketball," he said. "All you're really doing is priming the body and of course the mind to athletically perform. And the same thing can be done to speed up the rehab process."

Did you catch the rebound? Holder bounced when he used mindfulness and visualization to address his negative thoughts. He bounced again when he was re-injured and worked through, instead of denied, his disappointment—then moved on to take action toward his recovery.

FROM TRAUMA TO TRIUMPH

Many athletes report experiencing positive changes following their injuries. Sometimes this stress-related growth is a conscious choice (such as choosing to work on other areas of your performance not affected by the injury) and sometimes it's an outcome of the experience (in other words, reflecting on what you've learned about yourself).

Positive changes can include:

- Feelings of increased mental toughness
- Greater awareness of your body
- Greater perspective on the meaning of sport in your life, and a connection to a deeper motivation
- Feeling passion and gratitude for being able to participate and compete
- Increased understanding of the importance of recovery
- Bonding more closely with particular people, either within your sport or outside of it
- Increased empathy for teammates and competitors

- New mastery over technical aspects of your sport
- Returning to sport both mentally and physically stronger
- Bigger-picture view of your role in the sport—and perhaps an inclination toward leadership
- Ability to mentor and guide other athletes in ways that are incredibly satisfying
- A glimpse of a life after sport that is equally fulfilling and rewarding.

Some athletes, incredibly, ultimately express a degree of appreciation for what they've been through. Those we interviewed told us things like:

- "I'm not glad I went through it, but I'm glad I went through it." This was said by Adam Whiting, an international yoga instructor with a severe back injury that required surgery. "The biggest idea that I have taken away from this experience is simply gratitude for a body that is functional and relatively free from pain. I know that gratitude is often an overused cliché term, but I truly mean it."
- "This current injury is kicking my ass and it's really hard right now. But deep down, I really have to believe that it's honestly the best thing that could have happened to me, because it's forcing me to take a break that I never, ever, ever would have made myself take." This from Alia Gray, the elite marathoner with the sacral stress fracture who we introduced in Chapter 1. "In the long run, it could be the gift of a lot more healthy running years."
- "As crazy as it may sound, at the end of the day, I'm very, very grateful that I did deal with this because it brought me to where I'm standing today." Ashlee Groover, a collegiate softball player who had a hamstring tear, and who you'll meet in Chapter 6, said this.
- "Despite the challenges of my injuries, I am certain that my best physical and mental days are ahead—that being the best athlete I can ever be is only possible because of the challenges I face now." This was said by Hillary Allen, the trail runner from Chapter 1.

Even if you don't feel that way—if you aren't grateful for what happened, or if you would ultimately choose not to have coped with the injury, had you been able to make that choice—you can still harness the experience to propel you forward. Rob Jones describes this as "using the weight." Jones is a veteran who lost both his legs in an improvised explosive device (IED) blast in Afghanistan and who has gone on to complete incredible athletic feats, including winning a Paralympic bronze medal in rowing, riding a bike across America, and running thirty-one marathons in thirty-one cities in thirty-one days.

Jones described it this way in an interview: "Imagine everything that's stressing you is a weight on a barbell; you can either hold that stress or hold that weight until it weighs you down and you're pinned beneath it, or you can start shoulder pressing it or bench pressing it and putting it to use. The more you use it, the more you adapt to it and then the more you adapt to it, the easier it becomes to be able to handle that weight. Then you can handle more weight after that. It just kind of compounds on itself."

This process doesn't require you to be thankful or happy, he noted, merely that you accept reality and then act on it. In writing about it on his website, he noted that positive emotions do sometimes arise later in the process: "I can guarantee, however, you will ultimately be more thankful and happier that you used the hardship to your advantage than if you let it destroy you, and missed the opportunity to become more capable."

Finding a new purpose

During a weightlifting competition in January 2014, CrossFit athlete Kevin Ogar let a bar drop back behind him. It bounced against a weight stack and back against him, slamming into his spine with a force doctors told him was equivalent to a car traveling at seventy miles per hour. Surgeries on his back saved his life but not his function. Ogar was left paralyzed from the waist down.

Ogar undeniably faced some dark days after he got out of the hospital, when small things like the frustration of not being able to sit up without wobbling would send him into a near rage. Getting back to his sport as quickly as possible helped power him through. After just three weeks, he began lifting weights again.

A group of other adaptive athletes, dubbed "The Wheelchair Gang," welcomed him warmly; they hosted modified competitions called WheelWOD (CrossFit shorthand for Workout of the Day) that kept him engaged and motivated. (Learn how to find your own tribe with the Build Your Team drill on page 133.) Indeed, the entire CrossFit community rallied around him, hosting fundraisers, sending messages of support, and producing a documentary, *Will of Steel*, about his recovery and his efforts to join the CrossFit seminar staff, a challenge for even able-bodied athletes and coaches. (Setting a goal like this can prove powerful in your recovery—try the Grab Your Goals drill on pages 72–73.)

Today, he owns his own gym; travels the country as a Level 1 CrossFit coach; has helped build the organization's adaptive training program; and has even launched a new non-profit, The Reveille Project, that uses fitness to help returning veterans reintegrate into civilian life. He'd had the idea before he got hurt—but only afterward did he put it in motion.

"Really, it's a cliché, but everything in your life happens to you for a reason. You can choose to chase the reason or you can choose to retreat away from the reason that something happened to you; I think you have that choice," he said. "I don't know if I'd really change anything. I think this is exactly where I'm supposed to be."

Did you catch the rebound? Ogar bounced when he turned to The Wheelchair Gang for support and took part in their modified workouts. He bounced again when he used his injury as a motivator to fulfill his dreams: coaching at a high level, developing an adaptive training program, and starting a new non-profit.

JUST THE FACTS

- Injury is a common—almost universal—part of the athletic experience.
- You are entitled to your own unique injury journey.
- Injury poses many unknowns, and humans do not like uncertainty.
- Trauma—including injury—can inspire emotional and personal growth.
- Cultivating self-compassion offers you an objective perspective on your injury experience that enables you to keep moving forward.
- Athletes who have a high level of hardiness are more likely to experience stress-related growth.
- The progression of healing, both physically and mentally, is not going to be linear.
- Your response to trauma and the ups and downs of recovery can determine whether you have a miserable experience or a challenging, but ultimately rewarding, journey.

MENTAL SKILLS AND DRILLS

How can you navigate uncertainties like Tollefson did, practice self-compassion and hardiness like Holder, even—like Ogar—come to see serious setbacks as gifts? The following exercises will get you started down the path toward growth after injury.

MENTAL DRILL: GO FAR

*Feel, Accept, Recover—access your deeper emotions,
acknowledge them, and move on.*

Mental Skills:
Level 1, Rookie: Focus, Stress Management
Level 2, All-Star: Attitude, Emotional Intelligence, Self-Awareness
Level 3, Hall of Fame: Generosity, Mindfulness, Psychological
Flexibility, Resilience

People have a tendency to move away from uncomfortable feelings even though the best path to recovery is actually through them. Fighting against your feelings or suppressing them only makes them stick around longer, worsening the situation. Only when you allow yourself to really feel what you're feeling will you be able to accept where you're at and then take the next step forward.

Use the acronym FAR to remember the progression you need to go through: Feel, Accept, Recover.

- Feel: Label each emotion you are experiencing. You can refer back to the Emotion Decoder drill on pages 28–29, for example. Sit with that emotion for a moment, allowing it to merely exist.
- Accept: Once you hit on and really acknowledge and experience that specific feeling, you may naturally feel a release—that's acceptance, a settling into the truth. If it doesn't happen on its own, you can encourage it by thinking—or saying—a phrase like "I'd really prefer for things to be different, but this is the reality of where I am right now."
- Recover: Now that you've released the feeling and accepted reality, you can plot the next step toward where you want to go.

MENTAL DRILL: OBSTACLES TO OPPORTUNITIES

Think differently about setbacks to affect your reactions differently.

Mental Skills:
Level 1, Rookie: Focus
Level 2, All-Star: Attitude
Level 3, Hall of Fame: Discipline, Psychological Flexibility, Resilience

When you think about your injured status and your road to recovery, the language you choose to define your situation will impact how you feel, think, and react. For example, if you're approaching a specific rehabilitation exercise that you're not looking forward to and you think to yourself, "Ugh. This is gonna suck," you will now see and experience everything through that filter. If, instead, you can think of each challenge as an opportunity, you might even come to feel excited about figuring out the best way to approach it.

We can almost hear some of you groaning—"How am I supposed to look at a setback as an opportunity?" We know it isn't always easy. The good news is, you don't have to make that entire leap all at once, you can do it one step at a time. Instead of "This is going to suck," can you just think, "This is going to be hard"? Even that slight turn of phrase can make a significant difference in the way you feel about a situation. From there, you can move more easily to "This is going to be a challenge," and then, finally, to "This is going to be an opportunity."

Try completing a chart like the one below—there's a template in the workbook available at www.injuredathletesclub.com— with an obstacle of your own. Think about a potential obstacle or setback you are currently facing or that you might be facing in the future. Read each of the defining sentences below and for each sentence, write down the thoughts and emotions that immediately come to mind when you think about your situation through each filter.

DEFINING SENTENCE	EXAMPLE THOUGHTS	EXAMPLE EMOTIONS
This is going to **suck**.	I don't want to do this. I'm scared. It's going to hurt. I'm not ready.	Afraid. Annoyed.
This is going to be **hard**.	I don't know if I'm ready. Maybe I can ask them to put it off another week.	Fearful. Hesitant.
This is going to be a **challenge**.	I'm a little worried, but I know deep down I am ready and I can do this.	Concerned. Determined.
This is going to be an **opportunity**.	I get to do a new exercise. I'm so ready for this. I'm getting stronger.	Excited. Hopeful.

MENTAL DRILL: BAD NEWS/GOOD NEWS

*Practice holding two seemingly incompatible beliefs or emotions
at the same time and balancing them.*

Mental Skills:
Level 1, Rookie: Focus
Level 2, All-Star: Attitude
Level 3, Hall of Fame: Emotional Intelligence, Psychological Flexibility

Contrary to what we're told in TV commercials and social media quotes, *we aren't supposed to be happy all of the time.* We aren't supposed to be *anything* all of the time. However, sometimes you'll feel as if you've been hijacked by your emotions and that you've got stuck in them; as much as you want to feel differently, you're trapped. Unsticking yourself involves making sense of those moments when you're experiencing conflicting emotions.

For this mental drill, take any challenging situation and see if you can fill in the blanks to the following two sentences:

Well, the bad news is …

But the good news is …

For example: Well, the bad news is … I have to bow out of the race this weekend because my hamstring flared up. But the good news is … I'm going to get the chance to binge-watch my latest Netflix obsession.

Well, the bad news is … I'm not going to be able to take the field until my shoulder heals. But the good news is … I'll have more time to study tape and truly understand my role in critical plays.

Well, the bad news is … I may be looking at the end of my athletic career as I know it. But the good news is … I'll be able to help younger players from an experienced perspective.

This exercise helps you to hold on to the fact that it's OK to have conflicting emotions and that they can enable you to break out of feeling like the situation is all-or-nothing.

MENTAL DRILL: FUNHOUSE MIRROR

Identify common distortions in thinking so that you can begin to straighten them out.

Mental Skills:
Level 2, All-Star: Emotional Intelligence, Self-Awareness, Attitude
Level 3, Hall of Fame: Psychological Flexibility

When you go to the county fair or the carnival, the funhouse mirrors are a steadfast attraction. Stand in front of one mirror, and you have a giant skinny torso and no legs. Stand in front of another mirror, and you have long legs and a wavy head. The image is still you, but a false version of yourself—and of course these days you don't have to go to the carnival to experience this because there are apps and filters to do that for you in the comfort of your own home!

When injured, we can sometimes fall into distorted thinking patterns. These cognitive distortions are ways in which our brain interprets events wrongly and convinces us of things that might not be true.

When you have a thought, ask yourself: Am I seeing this through a regular mirror or through a funhouse mirror? If you catch yourself having a thought that's being distorted through the funhouse mirror, see if you can change it to reflect a more accurate interpretation. Use the chart below to assess your thoughts and identify if any of them are being viewed through the funhouse mirror.

DISTORTION	DESCRIPTION	EXAMPLE	MORE ACCURATE REFLECTION
All-or-nothing	Everything is black and white, there is no in-between. Anytime you say the words "always" and "never," you're probably engaging in all-or-nothing thinking.	"I *always* get hurt—my teammates never do."	I've dealt with a number of injuries this year. Some of my teammates have had better luck, but others have had their own struggles, too.
Maximize or minimize	Making things bigger or smaller than they actually are. Any time you exaggerate or downplay the circumstances of your situation, you are probably teetering on this type of thinking.	"I didn't really care about that race anyway." "This ankle sprain is the worst thing that's ever happened to me."	"I know racing would make my injury worse—but I'm still disappointed to sit out." "Spraining my ankle right now really sucks, but I know I can overcome it."
Personalization	When you engage in personalization, you are taking on all of the blame for something that is actually out of your control. You see yourself as the sole cause of this negative circumstance in your life. Guilt and shame are often indicators of this type of thinking.	"This wouldn't have happened if I were a better athlete."	"Every athlete—even the best ones—sometimes gets hurt."

DISTORTION	DESCRIPTION	EXAMPLE	MORE ACCURATE REFLECTION
Overgeneralizing	You see one negative event as throwing a wet blanket over your entire life. If one thing goes wrong, then everything goes wrong. If one aspect of your life is bad, everything in your life is bad.	"Missing this meet means I'll never get recruited. My friends and teammates are going to forget me, and I'll never go anywhere in life."	"There will be some recruiters at this meet, and it sucks to miss it. But my friends and teammates care about me and are supporting me. And I'll meet more recruiters at later meets."
Should and shouldn't	Sometimes we make up rules about how we think things "should" or "shouldn't" be, as if we've been handed a playbook that's carved in stone and we can't stray from the rules because they're right there in the stone playbook. Except they aren't.	"My knee shouldn't hurt after therapy. I'm therefore definitely not making progress. Back to square one."	"My knee hurts after therapy and it usually doesn't. I'm going to ask my trainer or physical therapist if that's normal or if we should adjust something about my program."
Jumping to conclusions	Also known as "fortune telling" and "mind reading," this type of thinking means you are concluding something about a situation on the basis of assumptions rather than facts. You assume the worst even though you don't necessarily have factual support for that conclusion.	"Coach didn't ask me how I was doing after practice. That means she thinks I'm a lost cause."	"Coach didn't check in with me like she usually does. I'm going to fill her in on how my therapy's going—and also ask how her life is going, because she seems a little distracted."

MENTAL DRILL: RECOVERY PERFORMANCE PROFILE

Rank yourself on the skills that are essential to your recovery.

Mental Skills:
Level 1, Rookie: Goal-Setting, Motivation
Level 2, All-Star: Self-Awareness

A Performance Profile is a popular sport psychology tool that is used to help athletes identify and assess skills that are important to their success as an athlete. Since your route back to peak performance goes through rehab right now, it's time to assess what skills are essential to your successful recovery. Once you have identified the skills that are important, you then rank yourself on a scale of one to ten regarding your ability in each skill. This exercise can help you celebrate your strengths and identify goals for improvement (more on that in Chapter 3).

Your profile does not represent any kind of judgment about you and your progress—when filled out honestly, it simply contains important information about your current status. It's subjective, so don't overthink it. Consider both mental and physical skills. You can even check with your coach, physical therapist, or athletic trainer to see if they would add anything to the list. Once you have ranked your ability in each skill you can shade in the appropriate areas and use the bar graph to have a visual representation of where you rank in the skills you need to develop to recover successfully. There's a template in the workbook at www.injuredathletesclub.com.

RECOVERY SKILL	1	2	3	4	5	6	7	8	9	10
Motivation										
Range of motion in knee										
Stress management										

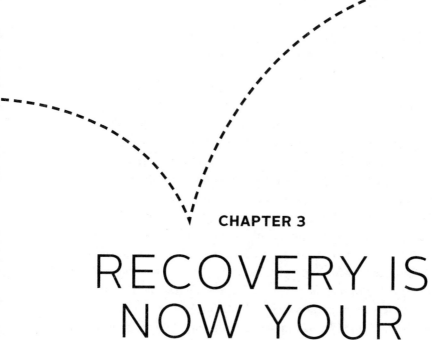

CHAPTER 3

RECOVERY IS NOW YOUR SPORT

"My greatest source of strength when the chips were down was applying principles from a previously active, athletic life to a recovery process without frustration that I couldn't train or wasn't racing."
—*Triathlete Fiona Ford*

Before you got hurt, you had goals: Run your fastest marathon, win a state title, earn the coveted spot on an Olympic team. Those ambitions kept you driven when you were at the peak of your performance, and one of the most challenging aspects of injury is watching them slip through your fingers. Though it's often hard to wrap your head around this when it first happens, you can tap into the very same drive during your recovery process by creating new goals and timelines. In being injured, you may have followed a path you didn't intend to follow and your destination may not even be exactly the same as it was before, but ultimately, you are still on an athletic journey.

One step at a time

The day after her crash, doctors matter-of-factly told British triathlete Fiona Ford her marathoning days were likely behind her. On June 23, 2012, she was riding back home from a fifty-mile training ride in the picturesque Surrey Hills when a car pulled out into a busy intersection. She and her bike both went flying. The impact of landing cracked her helmet, ripped the bike from under her, snapped her collarbone, fractured her sacrum and several vertebrae, and shattered her pelvis.

As she healed, Ford applied the same diligence to her rehabilitation that had made her a two-time world champion triathlete. The goals stayed small for a while. The first day, she was thrilled to wiggle her toes. A few days later, she focused on shuffling the distance of three feet from her hospital bed to the door. (It took twenty minutes, more than three minutes longer than her personal-best 5K time.) By the time she went home, ten days later, she had mastered crutching well enough to climb the thirteen steps into her apartment. (Use the Redefine Success drill on page 70 to identify your own rehab victories.)

Ford built the same type of structure into her days that she'd used when training, replacing runs with walks, swims with hydrotherapy, strength sessions with rehab work. Her detailed training log included notes on things like doctors' appointments, pain levels, and surgeries. Sure, she was using different metrics such as moments of mobility instead of those of distance, wattage, or heart-rate intensity—but if she tracked them, she could easily see how she was making progress. (Learn how to set—and measure movement toward—your own new targets in the Grab Your Goals exercise on pages 72–73.)

When Ford encountered a setback, she didn't panic, but instead evaluated what went wrong and addressed it. (You can learn to predict these situations in advance using the Plan B exercise on pages 181–182.) For instance, although she went back to coaching swimming—from a seat on the pool deck—for the first time a month after her accident, she found herself exhausted and in extreme pain for days afterward. Recognizing that she'd overreached, she waited about a week before trying again—and built in extra recovery time afterward.

At first, Ford didn't obsess about the idea of competing again. Slowly but steadily, she regained her ability to swim and cycle, then run. At the last minute, she lined up at the starting line of the Windsor Triathlon in the summer of 2015. She led her age group from the moment the gun went off until she broke the tape at the finish, winning it by twelve minutes and placing seventh overall. Next she tried a half Ironman in Barcelona, then Ironman Maastricht; even though she broke her toe coming out of the swim, she did well enough to qualify for the Ironman World Championships in Kona, Hawaii, that October.

As she neared the final mile of the 140.6 miles she'd covered in Hawaii that day—Ironman features a 2.4-mile swim, a 112-mile bike, and a 26.2-mile marathon—a man on a bike tracking a different athlete told her she'd passed enough women in her age group to earn a podium spot if she maintained her pace. "The penny dropped on the enormity of what I just delivered on that day. As I headed to the finish line, I can't tell you what the emotions were, it was just phenomenal," Ford said. At the age of forty-six, she finished in 10:46:53—about two minutes faster than she'd completed the same course nine years previously—and placed third among women age forty-five to forty-nine. "It has totally redefined, in my mind, what's possible for anyone." (She'd clearly cast herself as a character in her own Hero's Journey—learn to craft your own on pages 74–75.)

Did you catch the rebound? Ford bounced when she focused on small goals, such as wiggling her toes. She bounced again when she set up her rehab schedule to be just like her old training schedule, making recovery her new top priority.

One of the most severe consequences of injury is the loss of identity, the sense that you're adrift and purposeless without the training or competition to which you're accustomed. As you contemplate your shifted circumstances, this chapter will explain why it is you feel so unmoored—and will offer you guidance on how to redirect yourself, defining new goals and truly relishing their achievement. We'll pull back the curtain on the sometimes subconscious processes athletes go through in deciding how to proceed after an injury. And you'll come to understand how goals you don't even know you have can trap you in a cycle of fear and frustration—and learn how to break free.

It's possible to reframe your circumstances, to apply the very same athletic identity and approach you used in training and competition to recovering from your injury. Doing this can often allow you to regain much of your previous skill, abilities, and functionality, or even to surpass your past performances. Remember: *You are still an athlete, and your recovery is now your sport.* It's an idea that seems simple—but it has the power to restore the sense of purpose to your life.

CHARTING A NEW COURSE

Centuries ago, before the invention of the compass, before radar, before you could simply plug an address into Google Maps on your iPhone, explorers traveling by sea figured out which way to direct their sails by looking up into the sky and finding the North Star. Once they spotted the bright, shining glow of Polaris, they had their bearings; they were no longer lost. They knew which direction to steer the ship.

As an injured athlete, it's common to feel like you've lost your North Star. You simply don't feel like an athlete anymore—and therefore, you're unsure how to navigate the world around you. How do you approach each day? It's not clear how to fill the hours that used to be consumed by conditioning, strength training, practice, and competing. You've likely had to put the major goals that once consumed you on hold, sometimes for an uncertain length of time.

Research shows us that one of the biggest challenges you'll face as an injured athlete is dealing with the feeling that you have lost a part of yourself and your identity. At times it can feel like you've been completely cast aside. You're sidelined, and therefore must acquiesce and wait it out until you are capable of producing, able to use your body athletically again. Even if you're still training or participating in some capacity, it's likely that you'll be unable to perform at your peak, an experience that can be just as threatening to your concept of yourself as not being able to play at all.

This, in turn, can change your entire idea of who you are and what you have to offer the world. As you've likely already realized, the emotional shifts that come with injury can affect your life far beyond the gym, court, field, or track.

DON'T STOP NOW, GOAL-GETTER

Simply understanding the fact that you're still an athlete, just one at a different point in time, has tremendous power. But, of course, there's a lot more you can do to put this notion into practice. The first step is to let go of your old goals and create new ones.

Sometimes this is part of your grieving process—letting go of what you originally hoped and dreamed you'd accomplish, or at least letting go of the timeline along which you'd planned to do so. The Go FAR exercise at the end of Chapter 2 allows you to release your previous goals and expectations, truly giving yourself the opportunity to achieve new ones. Consciously adjusting your goals and shifting your focus to your optimal physical and mental recovery helps you find your North Star again, reassuring you that you are no longer lost.

The Grab Your Goals exercise at the end of this chapter will help you hone in on your specific goals. Examples might include:

◆ goals for your physical rehabilitation, such as spending a certain amount of time completing your exercises
◆ mental training goals, such as daily mindfulness or meditation training or practicing visualization
◆ lifestyle goals that can affect recovery and performance—say, sleeping more or changing your diet
◆ increasing your knowledge of the game or sport by reading, studying footage, or attending clinics or practices
◆ new performance or competition goals that take into account the probable timeline for your recovery (best set with input from your medical and coaching team).

Before you even get to the nitty-gritty of setting your new goals, it's helpful to understand some broad concepts. A goal needs to identify what you want to achieve and how you're going to achieve it, and getting there requires an effective goal-setting strategy. Clearly, defining your targets will help you direct your energy and efforts, keep you involved in your progress, and turn your focus toward aspects of your recovery that are in your control. Again, it might seem hard to believe at first, but following these principles can make your new goals just as meaningful—if not even more inspirational and rewarding—than the ones you've had to release.

To follow the rules of good goal-setting:

◆ Be specific
◆ Create accountability
◆ Continue fine-tuning
◆ Identify obstacles
◆ Celebrate accomplishments.

BE SPECIFIC

As a finely tuned athlete, you need more than general intentions—the more specific you are with your goals, the more likely you are to achieve them. Describing exactly what you are trying to accomplish, giving yourself a timeline for when you want to accomplish it, and having a game plan for how you're going to do it are all good ways to get specific—covering the what, when, and how. If you're too general with your goals, then you'll still be a bit afloat, with no map, process, or timeline. Often, people feel they're failing at their goals when, actually, they've simply overlooked this part of the goal-setting strategy.

ATHLETE EXAMPLE

CrossFit athlete Miranda Alcaraz was specific about her goals when she was rehabbing from two major injuries—a car accident that broke her neck in 2014, then an ACL tear during the CrossFit Games in 2015. Alcaraz knew her physical recovery, not to mention her state of mind, would be dramatically improved if she kept moving her body. At the point at which she left the hospital after surgery on her neck, doctors were hesitant to allow her to train at all at first. But once she showed them what she meant by air-squatting and how stable she stayed when lunging, they gave her the go-ahead.

Alcaraz built herself a schedule that started where she was and progressed slowly. At first, she'd do air squats, ride the bike, and drag a weighted sled around the gym. As soon as it was safe, she moved up to squatting an empty bar and lifting thirty-five-pound weights. The next week, she told herself, she could progress to forty pounds. Her strategy paid off: the year after her broken neck, she went back to CrossFit's Northern California Regional and placed seventh— the same ranking she'd achieved the year before.

CREATE ACCOUNTABILITY

When you're healthy, your coach might review your training log, and your teammates certainly know when you do and don't show up for practice. Anything you can do to recreate this type of accountability when you're injured will help you achieve your new goals. Some of this occurs naturally if you're working with an athletic trainer, physical therapist, or other medical professional—but still, you'll have plenty of work to do on your own.

How can you build some of this reinforcement and responsibility into your rehab? Some ideas:

◆ Sharing your goals, either verbally or on social media
◆ Writing them down in a journal or log
◆ Tracking your progress toward them
◆ Recruiting a goal buddy.

ATHLETE EXAMPLE

Chicago runner and coach Shawna Carter was already using the goal-buddy strategy pre-injury—she had a friend she had met up with at 6 a.m. every Wednesday for personal training sessions for years, a commitment she felt made her a better athlete. When Carter developed a sacral stress fracture, then a torn meniscus, she began to sink into depression and missed a few of their appointments. Her friend noticed—and asked her to come back, reminding Carter of how motivating their meetups had been for both of them. Her words were a big confidence boost during a low moment, and got Carter back to the gym and invested in her rehab.

CONTINUE FINE-TUNING

Setbacks are an inevitable part of any goal path, but especially so for goals related to injury recovery. The trajectory of your physical and mental recovery will not move forever in an upward linear path. There will be ups and downs; the ability to recognize these moments and adjust your goals is an essential skill to have.

Try not to think of your goals in terms of all-or-nothing, or that changing them in the face of new information or experiences means you have failed. Adjusting your goal is a normal and essential part of the process. The risk in not modifying your goals is that you give up on the goal altogether, or that you push too hard because you're being stubborn, insisting on staying on the original course—and end up setting yourself back further. Neither of these is worth the risk.

ATHLETE EXAMPLE

Ultrarunner Kevin Goldberg is another athlete who had to learn to alter his targets and timelines in deference to his body. In 2014, after training for a 100-mile ultramarathon and some ambitious adventures in fastpacking—a hybrid between backpacking and mountain running—he learned he had a congenital hip condition that would require two surgeries (one on each side) if he wanted to continue training and racing. He underwent the first in October 2016 and the second in January 2017. As he came back, he set lofty goals, putting races on his calendar long before he knew whether he'd be ready for them. He told his physical therapist about his aims, and she worked with him as best she could.

"A lot of them I didn't get to do, which didn't end up bothering me because of what I was able to do," he said. "But if I had known I wasn't going to be able to do them when I was planning them, I think I would have been crushed."

Not everyone will feel this way, of course—some might want to set goals that are more realistic and less likely to require major adjustments. But the important thing is to recognize what motivates you—and know that continuously updating your goals to better align with the rate at which you're actually improving will make you both happier and more successful in the long run.

IDENTIFY OBSTACLES

As we've just discussed, the path to your new goals isn't always smooth and clear; you might encounter some choppy waves or fog. If you think through your route ahead of time, it's likely that you can predict many of the potential obstacles that could interfere with your ability to accomplish these goals. Don't stop there, though—for each obstacle, come up with a game plan for how you want to respond, should it arise. Planning ahead in this way actually primes your nervous system to respond with less alarm and more confidence should you hit that particular bump in the road, enabling you to seamlessly implement the plan.

Psychologists call this technique "mental contrasting." If you've thought through—and perhaps even visualized—your responses in advance, your future self won't have to spend time worrying and figuring out what to do while in a highly emotional state. You already know exactly how you'll react to the situation. You can practice this technique with the Plan B drill on pages 181–182.

ATHLETE EXAMPLE

Joe Holder, the University of Pennsylvania football player turned coach and trainer we met in Chapter 2, employed mental contrasting in his recovery from a broken leg during his senior year. If he had a doctor's appointment to gauge his progress, for example, he'd imagine the best possible outcome—that he's cleared to run and practice again—as well as a more challenging one (that he needs another week or month of healing). In the latter case, he sees himself calmly feeling the disappointment, but then moving on to adjust the timeline and plan to accommodate this new information.

Once he was cleared to return to play, Holder employed a similar technique. Before he set out on a run, he imagined proceeding pain-free, with a smooth, strong stride. But he also pictured a run in which he felt an ache in his knee. In his mind, he might slow down or stop, ice the knee, and take a bit longer to recover before trying again—perhaps aiming for a shorter distance. Or he might envision continuing to run with a small amount of pain that doesn't worsen. What he doesn't picture is a scenario where the pain sends him on a spiral of despair and doubt, questioning whether he's set himself back or if he'll ever return to the field again.

CELEBRATE ACCOMPLISHMENTS

When you achieve a major goal in your athletic career, the celebration comes almost naturally—you receive glowing headlines, congratulations from your family and teammates, a ticker-tape parade, a chance to compete at the next level. One key to making your adjusted goals post-injury feel just as significant, so that you're equally driven to achieve them, is to make sure you're really reveling in your triumphs.

Each time you achieve one of your new goals, tell your athletic trainer or physical therapist how proud you are, whether the step you've reached is getting back on a bike or just getting through a tough set of exercises. Share your success with your teammates, post it on social media (you can share it in The Injured Athletes Club on Facebook), or mark it with a gold star in your training and rehab log. Do whatever it takes to make you feel like you've really and truly accomplished something special.

ATHLETE EXAMPLE

Triathlete Fiona Ford, whom we met at the beginning of this chapter, planned trips to warmer climes during the winter as she recovered from her crash. For one thing, this gave her specific, measurable targets to aim for—she knew she'd have to complete enough rehab to be able to sit comfortably on a plane for hours and drag a suitcase through the terminal. Once she reached her destination, she pampered herself, enjoying spa treatments, walks on the beach, and delicious meals.

Climber Jennifer Nicely, whom we'll meet in Chapter 4, nearly lost her arm when she fell while bouldering. She had mini-parties to celebrate various markers of her progress—namely, when she could tie her shoes, zip her pants, and braid her hair again. "You have to celebrate the small successes because they matter so much and you need to give yourself that space so you're embracing every step along the way. That's how your recovery can be as meaningful as possible, mentally and physically."

Now that you understand the fundamentals of good goal-setting, you can start thinking about your new targets. Once you narrow them down—using Grab Your Goals and the other drills at the end of this chapter—you'll begin finding your true north again. Your North Star is still there, but the conditions have changed, and you have to adapt. It can be hard for your ego, which responds to your more primal urges, to make this shift, as it wants to continue to gauge your feelings of success (and failure) in relation to your original destination, the original course you set. It's up to your higher brain to redefine what it means to be successful and adjust your goals accordingly.

PSSST ... DO YOU HAVE A SECRET?

Goals are good—but if you study them more closely, you might find some classified information buried within them. These are called *secret goals*, and they have the potential to sink your best plans and intentions, sometimes without you even realizing what's happening.

If you've been through an injury before, everything may be in clear view. You might be in a place where you know you need to feel your feelings, do the work, stick to your rehabilitation plan, and stay patient. You know that sometimes sustaining and recovering from injury is an inevitable part of being an athlete, and you accept your circumstances and your recovery timeline.

But in other cases, secret goals lurk in the shadows. They're separate from your stated goals, which are the ones you've defined with your coach or athletic trainer, the ones you write down on your Grab Your Goals worksheet. Your secret goals are known only to you, or perhaps to a few other trusted souls as well. For example, if your medical team tells you the recovery for your injury should take twelve to eighteen weeks, your stated goal might be to come back healthy in eighteen weeks, but your secret goal might be to come back in eleven weeks so that you can compete in a game or race that's really important to you, or in one where you feel like your team is counting on you.

Now, the goal itself isn't really the problem—indeed, sometimes ambitious aims can fuel us. The harm comes when you don't acknowledge or understand those secret goals and the effect they may have on your progress and your emotions, especially when you think about *not* accomplishing them.

Secret goals can sometimes cause athletes to overdo it during recovery, adopting the philosophy of, "Well, if this routine is good, that means more of it is better." You might do additional physical activities and exercises on top of what has been recommended, or push through pain when you shouldn't. While you can fool yourself into thinking this makes you a tough athlete, injury teaches us otherwise. *Sometimes a true sign of mental toughness is* not *pushing through—it's having the discipline to stop.*

Remember: *You'll never recover as quickly as you want to because you don't want to be injured in the first place.* Try to be patient. Secret goals can cause you to push too hard when your body (or your mind!) is not ready to.

Another potential effect of your secret goal is that it could leave you feeling discouraged and cause discord between you and your healthcare team. Imagine you've had a big discussion about goals, and you're improving along the timeline you and your trainer or therapist predicted—maybe even a little bit faster—but not quite swiftly enough to achieve your secret goal. The people working with you will be thrilled, but your response will be muted, even disappointed. This dissonance makes it difficult for you to accept and celebrate the goals you have accomplished, and also separates you from the rest of your team—when the reality is that you and your team function best when you're all working in tandem toward the same objectives.

If you're making progress but consistently feeling disappointed, ask yourself if you have a secret goal that you're not even admitting to yourself. If you know you have a secret goal you're afraid to tell people about, ask yourself why. Do you feel the goal is actually unrealistic, and are you afraid of having that fact mirrored back to you? Or is it actually realistic, but you're afraid to tell people because you fear what they'll think if you fail? If your secret goal makes you feel excited and drives you to stick to your rehabilitation program, it might be powerful to hold on to your secret goal in the knowledge that you might have to adjust your timeline depending on your progress. If your secret goal is not realistic and makes you feel that if you don't attain it, you're going to be a failure, consider getting rid of that goal and accepting that your stated goal *is a worthy goal*. In other words, pull your secret goals out into the light—and either commit to them or destroy them.

STICKING TO YOUR PLAN

OK, so you've got a new set of goals. In the best-case scenario, you've got a top-notch medical team working with you on a plan to achieve them. (We know that's not always the case—and we'll talk a little bit more about that in a minute, as well as offering more guidance on navigating the medical system in Chapter 6.) Once you have a solid rehabilitation plan, research shows that your odds of successfully recovering from your injury are much higher if you then stick to that plan.

Experts call this adherence—a fancy word for following your treatment and recovery protocol as it has been prescribed. Athletes who either don't do what's on their plan or are so eager and ambitious that they actually do *more* than what's on their plan may be undermining their own efforts, dragging out their healing process, and delaying their recovery and return to their sport. In fact, adherence is one of the most significant factors influencing your ability to rebound.

You might be thinking: "Well, I'm an athlete, of course I'm going to stick to my plan, so I can come back as soon as possible!" But actually, research shows that athletes aren't any better at this thing called adherence than people who don't participate in sports. There are plenty of reasons athletes don't stick to their plans—some psychological, some physical and logistical, and others that have to do with their relationship to the people around them. For example, you might be less likely to follow through if:

- You have low pain tolerance
- You're going it alone, as opposed to working in person with a physical therapist or athletic trainer
- You don't believe your treatment plan will work
- You don't believe you can do the exercises
- You're not self-motivated
- You lack a good social support network
- The logistics of scheduling rehabilitation and appointments seem onerous
- You question the value of your efforts
- You feel discouraged or that you're not seeing progress
- You lack clear goals or a sense of your role in the steps necessary for recovery
- You were already feeling burned out in your sport before your injury.

When you're injured and dealing with the prospect of time off and rehab, you conduct—sometimes without even realizing it—an assessment of the threats and benefits of following through with your recovery plan. It's the outcome of this assessment that determines, in large part, whether or not you will stick to your plan—and therefore, how successfully you will recover. And you continue to go through this process, over and over, as your recovery continues. Recognizing that this is happening, understanding where you might be getting stuck, and learning what steps to take to either resolve your conflicts or release them frees you to move forward. Use the following guide to help you determine where you're getting hung up, and how to break free.

THOUGHTS THAT TELL YOU YOU'RE STUCK

- "It's not really that bad—it'll probably heal on its own."
- "I know what to do. I don't really need to go to the doctor."
- "I'm tough enough to handle a little pain; I don't need to do anything."

WHAT YOU'RE ASSESSING (WHETHER YOU REALIZE IT OR NOT):
- How severe is my injury?

HOW TO GET UN-STUCK

If your pain or decreased function persists even after you scale back or rest, or if it's interfering with your gait or the way you perform your sport, it's probably time to seek some expert attention. You might hear that there's a relatively easy way to address your injury that doesn't involve time away from training or competition. Even if the news is bad, it's better to hear that sooner and avoid worsening the situation. Ask your medical team to explain simply and clearly how serious your injury is, and what might happen if you don't follow your protocol. Online research can help here too, provided it's from credible sources—though with the caveat that it's not going to be as specific to YOU (remember, as we told you in Chapter 2, you're special) as a personal medical opinion.

THOUGHTS THAT TELL YOU YOU'RE STUCK

- "Is this really going to help me get back to my sport?"
- "My doctor's not an athlete, so I'm not sure if this is the right treatment plan for me."
- "This doctor doesn't really know his/her stuff."
- "My doctor's more interested in money or in just getting me out of the room—we don't have the same goals."

WHAT YOU'RE ASSESSING (WHETHER YOU REALIZE IT OR NOT)
- Do I believe this will help?

HOW TO GET UN-STUCK

If you trust your medical team but not your plan, ask your doctors for details about how each part of the plan connects to your goals and recovery. If you don't trust your team, evaluate the possibility of finding new providers. (We know that's not always possible—refer to Chapter 6 for ways to build a better support team.)

THOUGHTS THAT TELL YOU YOU'RE STUCK

- "My body is not really ready for this."
- "I don't trust my [knee, ankle, elbow, other injured body part] to be able to do this."
- "This is gonna hurt, and I'm scared—I don't know if I can handle the pain."

WHAT YOU'RE ASSESSING (WHETHER YOU REALIZE IT OR NOT)

◈ Do I believe in my ability to work through the recovery plan?

HOW TO GET UN-STUCK

First, recognize exactly what makes you anxious, and take steps to address it (the Anxiety Pyramid at the end of Chapter 5 can help). Use the Pain Log, also in Chapter 5, to monitor your pain and determine when it's at a manageable level and when it's so severe you need to pull back. And realize that even if you push a little too far and have to dial things back, you're not heading back to square one. In fact, you're still ahead of the game, because you have new information about your current capabilities and limitations and how to move forward safely.

THOUGHTS THAT TELL YOU YOU'RE STUCK

◈ "This [icing, stretching, rolling, rehab exercise] isn't really that big of a deal. It's not going to set me back if I skip it."
◈ "Eh, I'm not really going to make things worse if I just go to bed instead of stretching first."
◈ "I'm busy so I'm going to skip rehab—skipping it won't really affect my healing process."

WHAT YOU'RE ASSESSING (WHETHER YOU REALIZE IT OR NOT)

◈ Am I likely to sustain further harm if I skip the rehabilitation exercises?

HOW TO GET UN-STUCK

Do some research—either on your own or with your medical team—into how each element of your plan contributes to your recovery. Use the Thoughtstopper exercise at the end of Chapter 7 to defuse negative reactions when they arise.

Note that not following your plan doesn't mean you're a bad patient, a terrible person, or an unworthy athlete. In general, however, adherence does play a key role in successful recovery. So if you're skipping out on your appointments or exercises and finding reasons to do anything but what your doctor, physical therapist, or trainer told you to do, you might be holding yourself back. Doing a little detective work as to why your motivation is wavering can help you stay on track. Sometimes simply recognizing the thoughts that stand between you and doing those hip exercises or knee extensions takes away the power of those thoughts; in other cases, taking action on your part can resolve any conflicts that may have arisen.

You do not have to be a passive participant on this injury journey. You do not have to just "sit this out." Holding on to your athletic mindset and directing all the energy and resources you had been putting into practice and competition toward your recovery and return to sport allows you to see the opportunity in injury. If you take this attitude, you can truly start to get excited about your new goals and the plan you'll put in place to achieve them.

Defined by resilience

The five ACL tears Jacki Gemelos sustained during her six years on the USC basketball team certainly threatened to rob her of her athletic identity, and more. The constant cycle of re-injury and rehab left her so worn down it began to drain her overall confidence as a person, making her shy and closed-off.

After the third surgery—not to mention the fourth and the fifth— Gemelos certainly contemplated walking away. But her love for the game ran deep, and she knew her career wasn't over. She'd think about her father, Steve Gemelos, who had played basketball in college and for two years as a pro in Greece, and about the deep bond they shared from their years of going to tournaments and practices together.

Each time she'd have the surgery, she'd then go through the rehab her doctors, athletic trainers, and coaches recommended. Her fifth time, she started seeing a new physical therapist, who infused her routine with fresh energy and a holistic approach to her recovery. Her knees locked straight when she landed, he noticed; she'd repeatedly hyperextend them, putting her tendons at risk. So, as she regained strength and function after surgery, she worked on landing with her knees slightly bent—an entirely new goal for her to target that would eventually pay dividends in years of injury-free playing.

Although going to practice when she couldn't play sometimes pained her, Gemelos kept showing up. Soon, she noticed, her sideline view of the game gave her an advantage none of her teammates or competitors possessed. She could see where each player stood coming off a pick-and-roll or stagger screen, and would note the body positions that worked best in each defensive play. (Use the In/Out of Control drill on page 88 to find other skills to work on and the Performance Profile 2.0 drill on page 179 to quantify your newfound talents.)

When she finally returned to the court, Gemelos not only felt stronger physically, she also had a mental edge. "Before, I was always playing based off my talent and hard work. But being able to study the game and try to put it in that way, I could play with my head," she said. Gemelos went on to play a season for the Chicago Sky in the WNBA, and now plays in Italy.

Even after decades on the court, she knows she has much more to learn. But now she possesses a rare blend of athleticism and knowledge that has enabled her to extend her career and continue improving. She derives great satisfaction from mentoring and guiding younger athletes, especially through injuries. And perhaps most importantly, she said, she's moved far beyond her self-doubting past. "This series of injuries defined who I was as a person: someone who's resilient and has persevered through adversity. I've used that in every aspect of my life."

Did you catch the rebound? Gemelos bounced when she kept going to practice even when it was challenging to do so. She bounced again when she adopted the identity of a resilient person.

JUST THE FACTS

◆ You are still an athlete, and recovery is now your sport.
◆ Adherence to your treatment plan is one of the most significant factors influencing your ability to rebound.
◆ Defining new goals for your rehab creates momentum toward recovery.
◆ The more specific you are with your goals, the more likely you are to achieve them.
◆ Accountability creates commitment and motivation to reach your goals.
◆ Predicting the obstacles that may lie in your way and developing a game plan for how to respond in advance dramatically improves your ability to navigate them.

- You'll never recover as quickly as you want to because you don't want to be injured in the first place.
- You do not have to be a passive participant on this injury journey. You can apply all the energy and resources you had been putting into practice and competition toward your recovery and return to sport.

MENTAL SKILLS AND DRILLS

How can you adopt Ford's athletic approach to rehab, Gemelos' attitude of learning from your new perspective, Goldberg's ability to set and then adjust new goals, Alcaraz's step-by-step rebuilding plan? The following drills will help shift your mindset from one of victim or passive participant in recovery back to being the captain of the ship that is your athletic body, pointing toward the North Star that is your recovery.

(*Continues on page 70*)

MENTAL DRILL: REDEFINE SUCCESS

List and celebrate other ways to "win."

Mental Skills:
Level 1, Rookie: Confidence
Level 2, All-Star: Attitude
Level 3, Hall of Fame: Generosity, Psychological Flexibility

One of the many challenges in recovering from injury involves dealing with the temptation to define your current feelings of success in terms of what your body was capable of doing before you were injured. You might not have exactly the same goals now, but you can still find "wins" to celebrate, key milestones in your recovery. To get started with your celebration list, answer the following:

- What are your "firsts"? (For example, when you are weight-bearing again, when you can walk again, the first time you can throw, etc.)
- When are the times you've demonstrated perseverance and resilience?
- Who are the people you're grateful for?
- What are all of the things you are proud of?
- In what ways do you feel you are becoming stronger?

Also, come up with real ways of celebrating those wins—give yourself a special treat like a new piece of gear, post a social-media message, arrange a get-together (maybe with cake) with good friends. Make it truly feel like a worthwhile accomplishment, and you'll find you have even more motivation to go for the next goal.

MENTAL DRILL: INJURY MANTRAS

Brainstorm a list of phrases to pump yourself up during tough moments.

Mental Skills:
Level 1, Rookie: Stress Management
Level 2, All-Star: Attitude
Level 3, Hall of Fame: Generosity, Resilience

When you hit a setback during rehabilitation or if someone says something to you that's inadvertently hurtful, it can be helpful to have an anchor—something that keeps you grounded. Injury mantras provide just that in a word or phrase that guides you through your recovery, reminding you of your strength, resilience, and hope. Using a mantra is akin to planting the seed of a thought in your mind. As you repeat it, it starts to take root; as you live it, the seedling grows and sprouts leaves. Come up with an injury mantra that will serve as your anchor, the one word or phrase you can go to that will plant the thought seed that makes you feel calm, confident, and resolute.

- Every day I'm stronger.
- Strength, grace, resilience.
- There is a light at the end of this tunnel.
- I will persevere.

MENTAL DRILL: STOP/START/CONTINUE

Identify the helpful things you're already doing, new strategies to adopt, and self-sabotaging behaviors to leave behind.

Mental Skills:
Level 1, Rookie: Focus, Goal-Setting, Motivation
Level 2, All-Star: Self-Awareness
Level 3, Hall of Fame: Discipline

As humans, we are masters of sabotaging our own efforts even though we have the best of intentions. It can be meaningful to pause and reflect on the ways you might be holding yourself back as you proceed through your injury and recovery. For this drill, come up with at least three answers for each of the following questions; there's a blank form to complete in the workbook at www.injuredathletesclub.com. Once you finish, you will have some new goals!

QUESTIONS	EXAMPLES	YOUR ANSWERS
What do I need to STOP doing in order to recover successfully?	"I need to stop getting to bed late, since sleep is important in healing." "I need to stop comparing where I am right now with where I was before I got hurt."	
What do I need to START doing in order to recover successfully?	"I need to start icing on more of a regular basis." "I need to start meditating or visualizing my return to my sport."	
What do I need to CONTINUE doing in order to recover successfully?	"I need to continue doing my rehab exercises." "I need to continue building my support team" (see Chapter 6 for more on exactly how to do it).	

MENTAL DRILL: GRAB YOUR GOALS

Set new physical, mental, and motivational targets to shoot for during recovery.

Mental Skills:
Level 1, Rookie: Confidence, Focus, Goal-Setting, Motivation
Level 3, Hall of Fame: Discipline

Setting deliberate goals for your injury rehabilitation and recovery will help you shift your focus to something that's in your control, offer an opportunity to redefine success, motivate you to work on your rehabilitation, and boost your confidence as you see progress. Together with your rehabilitation team, identify targets you're working toward—or identify them on your own using an exercise like the previous one, Stop/Start/Continue. Then get specific with your goal-setting, writing out your objectives, a timeline, the resources and support you'll need, your strategy for accomplishing your goal, and how you will know if you are on the right track. Remember: *You are still an athlete, and recovery is now your sport.* Use the following template—you'll find a blank one in the workbook at www.injuredathletesclub.com—to write out your new athletic goals, and update them with new ones as you accomplish each set.

What's my objective?	
When do I want to have accomplished this goal?	
What supplies/resources/support do I need to accomplish this goal?	
What specific strategies will I employ to accomplish my goal?	
How will I know if I am on the right track with my progress?	

MENTAL DRILL: HEALING VISIONS

Use visualization to picture your body growing stronger.

Mental Skills:
Level 1, Rookie: Confidence
Level 2, All-Star: Visualization
Level 3, Hall of Fame: Mindfulness

There are many different ways to use visualization throughout your injury recovery, including visualizing the healing of your injury. Apps like Headspace offer guided meditations that make this visualization easy. You can also build your own using any of the scripts below. Practice it daily for about ten or twenty minutes. (Doing these practice sessions can even become one of your new goals.)

- For those who are scientifically minded: Research alone or with your medical team the physiology of your injury and the healing process. Imagine it unfolding as a series of time-lapse photographs— your bone fusing together, new muscle tissue growing, tendons restructuring.
- For a more holistic view: Imagine a warm light radiating from the place of your injury, and feeling the warmth of the light on your skin as the glow heals your injured body part.

MENTAL DRILL: HERO'S JOURNEY

Make your injury narrative that of a triumphant protagonist.

Mental Skills:
Level 1, Rookie: Motivation
Level 2, All-Star: Attitude
Level 3, Hall of Fame: Generosity, Psychological Flexibility, Resilience

Most stories have a beginning, a middle, and an end. Right now, you are smack dab in the middle of your own narrative. Some of the most exciting tales we grew up with involved a hero who has to rise to the occasion to meet challenges and save the day—think Frodo Baggins, Katniss Everdeen, Dorothy Gale, and Harry Potter. Author and mythologist Joseph Campbell described this archetypal story as "The Hero's Journey." If you've seen any of the movies featuring these heroes (*The Lord of the Rings*, *The Hunger Games*, *The Wizard of Oz*, or any of the Harry Potter movies) you'll know that often the "hero" is an underdog or an ordinary person like you and me—and that they follow a distinct path.

Now it's your turn to write your own Hero's Journey story within the context of your experience as an athlete. Answer each of the questions below up to the point where you feel like you are right now in your journey. Think about writing your story as if it will be adapted into a screenplay and turned into a multi-million-dollar film. What was your call to adventure, the thing that brought you into your sport? At what point did you "cross the threshold" from the world you were familiar with into the unknown? How do you see the story playing out? Have fun with it!

Call to Adventure: This is the call to action, the force that pulls you out of the mundane and familiar into adventure. What was your call to adventure?

Assistance: The hero needs help. Who gives you guidance that provides you with essential insight, information, and the tools necessary for your successful journey?

Crossing the Threshold: The departure. What symbolizes the moment you crossed the threshold and committed to the journey ahead?

Trials: The hero is tested. You are confronted with challenges and the progress of your journey is threatened. What obstacles are thrown in your path to test your skill and strength?

Crisis: During the crisis the biggest obstacle is faced. For the hero, this is the darkest hour. What is the biggest fear you had to face?

The Reward: You survive the crisis and emerge with a treasure gained from your journey. It can be a talisman, a new knowledge or understanding, or a goal accomplished. What gifts and rewards did you receive during your journey?

Transformation: You are changed, transformed by this experience. The person who completed this journey is not the same person who started it. How has this journey changed you? How are you a different person now from the person you were when you started this journey?

Return: The hero has succeeded and circles back to his or her familiar world once again. All the doubts have been quelled, and the enemies slain. How has your journey freed you?

MENTAL DRILL: YES, AND...

Adopt an improv-based approach to shifting your story.

Mental Skills:
Level 1, Rookie: Confidence
Level 2, All-Star: Attitude, Communication
Level 3, Hall of Fame: Discipline, Psychological Flexibility

As you reach milestones during your injury recovery, you might feel some internal conflict—excited because you are finally weight-bearing or because you just got cleared and are returning to certain aspects of your training, but also aware that you are far short of your pre-injury status. Remind yourself to gauge your current feelings of competence and success on the basis of your injury-recovery progress and not by comparing where you are now with where you were before you got injured.

When you are redefining success at this point, eliminate "Yeah, but..." from your story. Instead of "Yeah, but..." you need to switch to "Yes, and..." It's a trick improv actors have long used to keep creativity and collaboration flowing—saying "No" or "But" during a scene shuts your fellow actor down. Using "Yes, and..." instead builds everyone up and opens the door to new possibilities. (Note that this strategy not only makes you feel better, it also improves your interactions and relationships, which leads to a stronger support system!)

Someone says: "You ran a mile! That's awesome!" Instead of responding: "Yeah, but I used to run ten miles and my pace was a lot faster" try: "Yes, and I can't wait until I am up to two miles!"

Someone says: "Congrats on your first day back to practice! That's a huge milestone!" Instead of: "Yeah, but I'm probably not going to be able to compete by the start of the season" try: "Yes, and I can't wait to keep progressing and get back to competition!"

You might feel like you're "faking it" a bit at first. That's OK—the more you respond in this way, even if you have to consciously rephrase something after you've already said it, the more natural it will become.

CHAPTER 4

THE TIME-TRAVEL TRAP

"I wouldn't wish injury on anyone, and I would never want to go back through that process again. But in a weird way, I think it was probably the best thing that ever happened to me. I don't know what's next. But I know that right now, today, I feel fantastic."
—*Ultrarunner and obstacle course racer Amelia Boone*

One of the biggest challenges of injury is feeling there are so many aspects of your recovery that are out of your control. You can't command surgical wounds to mend or fractured metatarsals to fuse; nor can you dictate whether your doctor will call you back or whether your insurance will pay for your MRI; and you lack the ability to regulate (or even truly know) what your teammates say about you when you're not around. But while you can't turn back the clock or fast-forward your healing process, you do have more power than you realize, starting with the management of your own emotions and reactions in the present moment.

Moving beyond shame

Amelia Boone was confronted with a loss of control not once, but twice, when major injuries interrupted her previously triumphant running and obstacle-course racing career. She'd done her first obstacle course race—a Tough Mudder—almost on a whim in 2011. The next year, she won the second-ever World's Toughest Mudder, a 24-hour race studded with obstacles with names like "Ladder to Hell" and "Arctic Enema." From there, Boone ascended the podium at nearly every race she entered and won more than thirty of them, often beating all the men too.

Boone began dabbling in ultrarunning in 2016. In just her second race, a 100K, she took second place and earned her "golden ticket"—an automatic entry to the prestigious Western States Endurance Run, the world's oldest one hundred-mile trail race.

During a long training run about two months before the race, she felt a sharp pain in her quad. The next morning, when she tried to get out of bed, she crashed to the floor. An MRI revealed a stress fracture in the shaft of her femur. Not only would she not be able to run in the Western States two months later, she'd spend four weeks on crutches, and twelve weeks not running at all.

Her training and forward momentum halted, Boone felt angry and defensive. She'd done everything she was "supposed to," she thought, and still ended up sidelined. Other days, she rode what she calls the "merry-go-round of self-flagellation." She said in an interview with us, "Who runs enough to fracture their femur? It's kind of shameful in a way, because with stress injuries, you have no one else to blame except yourself."

Dwelling on the past hurt and looking ahead offered little reassurance. A runner update email she got from Western States less than a week later caused her to break down in tears, mourning the loss of the chance she'd had.

Boone didn't give herself time for much thoughtful contemplation. She traded the hours she'd spent getting lost on the trails by her house for swimming and one-legged push-ups, and crutched miles a day, until blisters formed on her hands. If recovery was now her sport, she aimed to climb the podium there, too. Though she outwardly told herself she'd take it slow and listen to her body, in reality she had secret goals (see Chapter 3 for more about those). What if, a tiny inner voice said, she could get back in time for the Spartan World Championships in Tahoe, two months after she got off crutches? And then defend her title at the World's Toughest Mudder a month after that?

Her body had other ideas. Four weeks after Boone came off crutches and three weeks after she'd started running again, she was diagnosed with a sacral stress fracture on the left side. That meant another twelve weeks of no impact, of no running. As she worked her way through the initial shock, tears, and pints of Ben & Jerry's, a friend posed a key question: Had she really, truly accepted the first injury? Boone had to admit she hadn't. She'd tried to maintain control and cross-train around her regrets and fears. She vowed to do things differently this time around. (Use the Stop/Start/Continue drill on page 71 to figure out thoughts and behaviors that might be hindering or helping your recovery.)

She started by forgiving the Amelia of the past, who had mistakenly believed she could make her body do anything she wanted, as long as her mind was willing. She now knew she couldn't control the amount of pounding her legs could handle or the speed at which her bones rebuilt. However, she did have agency over her emotions and reactions, not to mention her attitudes toward training and racing—and those things, she could change for the better. (The In/Out of Control drill on page 88 can help you differentiate between the factors which you can and can't influence.)

Boone stopped all activity—including biking, swimming, and cross-training—for a whole month, to let her body regenerate. She used the Calm app to meditate each night before bed (more on that and other apps in the Mindfulness Meditation drill on pages 89–90). She asked her support system to call her out when she fell into a spiral of self-blame. Step by step, mile by mile, she worked her way back to running, then racing. On April 29, 2017—almost a year to the day after her initial fracture—Boone won the Rodeo Beach Half Marathon. The next month, she was back to obstacle course racing, placing second at the Austin Super Spartan.

More importantly, Boone began feeling a sense of joy and peace with the sport—and with herself—that she'd never experienced before. She'd once cried before races, fearful no one would like or respect her if she failed to podium. Now, she lined up with joy, grateful for the opportunity and free to fail—or succeed—without regret. In March 2018 she even attempted the Barkley Marathons, a one hundred-mile race with no set course, extremely challenging conditions, and only fifteen finishers in its thirty-two-year history. She wasn't among them—no one finished that year—but she had reveled in the opportunity to try. She's faced additional injuries since, and each time learns a little bit more about her body and her mind. "What's funny is that, as tough as this injury cycle has been, I've never let go of the unwavering belief that my best running and racing days are still ahead," she wrote after another bone injury in 2019.

Did you catch the rebound? Boone bounced when she forgave herself and let go of the past. She bounced again when she used meditation and cues from her support team to continue staying mindful and positive.

YOUR BRAIN: A SELF-DRIVING TIME MACHINE

Our thoughts have a natural tendency to travel through time—moving into the past or into the future. Trouble is, your recovery is happening right here, in the present. Rewinding the tape to go back in time to before you were injured or fast forwarding it to the time when your injury has become just a memory can keep you from recognizing where you are in this moment and staying focused on what you need to do right now.

These journeys through time often feel completely out of your command—as though you have an automated time-travel device installed it in your gray matter. What's worse, the engineers seem to have pre-programmed the vehicle to take you back to the worst day of your life or take you forward to a depressing version of the future, not to the day you performed at your best or ahead to the celebration of your biggest victory.

Even when we do return to the present, the settings on the machine can seem stuck on "chaos" and "futility." Given that injury inherently means you're not where you want to be, it's easy and natural to focus on what's difficult and also on what's out of your hands. You can quickly lose hope and feel like nothing you do will have any effect on the outcome.

When you focus on the things you can't control about your situation, you end up having negative emotions and experiences. The following types of script have likely run through the head of pretty much every injured athlete, on repeat. See if you recognize them in your own thoughts and reactions:

- ◆ **Failures** pile up when you ruminate on what you can't alter about the past.
  - ○ If only I hadn't headed out for that run/reached for that ball/ pitched that last inning.
  - ○ Why did I let this happen?

- I wish my coach hadn't told me to make that play, or had taken me out of the game when he should have.
- If only my teammate or opponent hadn't screwed up or taken me down.
- What if I hadn't missed that game/race/competition—what would that have meant for my career?

◈ **Frustrations** occur when you dwell on what's out of your hands right now.
- This sucks.
- I can't believe I'm missing practice/the game tomorrow.
- My teammates are disappointed in me.
- I can't believe my coach took me out of the starting lineup.
- My sponsors are dropping me.
- I can't believe my perfect record is now blemished.
- My fans think I'm weak or unworthy.

◈ **Fears** arise when you think about what's unknown or uncertain about the future.
- I might not make it back in time for playoffs ...
- What if I don't come back as strong as I was before I was injured?
- What if the doctors can't fix me?
- My teammates might not trust me.
- I'm going to lose my starting spot.
- What if I get injured again?
- What if I can't come back at all?

It's completely normal to have these thoughts. Our brains are hard-wired to focus on the negative—it's part of what's enabled us to survive as a species. There's no way you can force your brain to stay present and positive all the time, and attempting to do so will merely cause more frustration. In Chapter 1, we talked a little bit about what happens when you bury or deny your emotions. When you do, you'll have a much harder time moving past them than if you truly own up to and experience them.

FLIPPING THE OVERRIDE SWITCH

You don't have to get stuck in the past wishing things had never happened, or stuck in the future, consumed with fears that hold you back. Nor must you stay suspended in an unchangeable version of the present, biding your time and feeling like you are in limbo, stuck in a waiting room until someone calls your number and your circumstances change.

For now at least, driverless cars must have a manual override switch, a panic button that can allow a trained human driver to take over. And here's a secret: Your time-traveling, negative-focused brain has a similar mechanism. You just have to step up to the controls. One of the most powerful mental skills you can have as an athlete, and as a human, is the ability to stay in the present moment—or, more specifically, the ability to *bring yourself back to the present moment*, and to do so without judgment. Though it's not quite as instantaneous as hitting a button or flipping a switch, we would argue that with dedication and practice, it's possible to come back to the present, drop the negative storylines spinning through your head, and trade the cycle of hopelessness, despair, and anxiety for positive forward momentum.

In fact, *you can turn the three negative Fs of Fear, Frustration, and Failure into three positive As in three simple steps*:

- **Accept:** Let go of what you can't control.
- **Adapt:** Change your reactions to what's happening.
- **Act:** Do what you can right now to create the best possible future.

Those three steps—Accept, Adapt, Act—don't always proceed in exactly that order, nor do they always only unfold once. As we've said before, recovery is rarely a linear process. However, that actually makes this framework even more reassuring. You can return to it any time you start to feel yourself losing your perspective or focus.

A new ascent

Climber Jennifer Nicely had fallen probably hundreds of times before while bouldering—climbing lower walls without ropes or harnesses. She always tumbled safely onto the crash pads underneath. But on April 4, 2012, she swung off the top of the boulder and landed before she had time to brace for the fall. The jolt not only dislocated the joint, it severed her muscles, tendons, and—most alarmingly—her brachial artery. She needed immediate surgery or she might lose her arm—and in fact, even with surgery, the doctors weren't entirely sure they could save it. Of course, Nicely was terrified—but she swiftly began to turn her Fs into As.

She *feared* the loss of her arm. But even as she was wheeled into surgery, she *accepted* the situation she was in: "I just knew that I needed to narrow focus. I wasn't going to be able to make sense of this and wasn't going to be able to control this moment as much as I wanted to, so I was only going to ask the questions I needed to know the answers to right then." She committed in advance to *adapting*, saying to herself, "I don't care if I have to do it with one arm, I'm going to climb again."

During rehab, instead of feeling *frustrated* by her slow progress, she *acted* to celebrate each milestone—relearning how to zip her pants, braid her hair, tie her shoes. Four and a half months later, she was climbing on ropes again; in 2015, she competed on *American Ninja Warrior*. Although it took her a few years to feel comfortable bouldering again, six years later she's back to the sport she loves.

She still sometimes *fears* another tumble, and flashes back to her fall—sensations that are triggered when she hears sirens come for other climbers, something that's happened twice at the gym since. But, she *accepts* that those feelings are part of her—sometimes heading to the bathroom to wait them out—then *adapts* by focusing on the positive emotions associated with the experience. For instance, she calls to mind the gratitude she felt for the medical team, the friends and family who rushed to the hospital and stayed by her as she recovered, and the strength she'd never known she possessed until it was so seriously tested.

THE MINDFUL TRAVELER

The past can inform you and the future can inspire you, but your power to take action only exists in the present moment. That's why mindfulness is so key to the **Accept, Adapt, Act** process. Mindfulness is the skill that can help you stay in— or bring yourself back to—the present moment, without judgment or blame, when your self-driving time-travel machine starts to steer your thoughts and emotions backward or forward in time. When you're mindful, you can recognize and become aware of what is happening in the present moment without being attached to it—essentially, you can become an observer of yourself.

Sometimes our decisions to travel into the past, present, or future are in an effort to avoid anxiety and other uncomfortable emotions. Again, though, the way to most effectively neutralize these negative emotions isn't to move away from them, it's to move through them. With mindfulness, you can essentially hold those feelings in your hand like an object, studying them. You can cultivate a desire to understand them rather than being attached to them, and by doing so, you strip them of their power to control you.

After all, you can have a thought without acting on it; you can have an emotion without attempting to alleviate or enhance it. Thoughts and emotions are fleeting. With mindfulness, you learn to tell yourself: "This is how I'm feeling right now, but that doesn't mean this is how I will always feel." If you are time-traveling, mindfulness can bring you into the present moment so that you can recognize how you're feeling, accept your circumstances (both physically and emotionally), and then shift your mindset and choose to make decisions based on your bigger goals instead of on the whims of your transitory thoughts and emotions.

Pathways to peace

In Chapter 2, we met Kirsten Cooper, who had a serious crash on the slopes in Chile while skiing for Team USA. Near the end of her athletic career, she began going to yoga classes with her mom, who was in the early stages of Alzheimer's disease and needed help getting into an exercise routine. The ritual proved healing for Cooper, too. She felt so at home on the mat that she continued practicing yoga even after she quit skiing, eventually becoming a teacher herself. Not only did her body feel better, yoga's focus on breathing and staying in the present moment slowly began calming her mind.

After her horrific crash, Cooper had raced in fear, then rushed to numb uncomfortable feelings with drugs, alcohol, and other risky behaviors. Today, practicing mindfulness has created enough space for her to calmly consider her reactions and adapt them, so when she encounters a difficult emotion, she doesn't immediately seek to numb it.

Now that she's retired from skiing and is a busy grad student in sport psychology, Cooper doesn't always get to practice yoga as much as she would like to. "But I try to live mindfully; eat mindfully, slowing myself down and feeding my body; I drive mindfully; walk mindfully; just be in that space with myself as often as I can," she said. For years, she'd paint her right thumbnail red as a reminder to slow down and refocus any racing thoughts. "Now I actually wear a bead bracelet on my right wrist. It clicks on things a lot, especially when I'm typing. That's the thing that jars me back into the present."

THE DAILY MINDFULNESS HABIT

Meditation is the most common way to practice and access mindfulness, and we'll have some suggestions on how to get started in the Mental Skills & Drills section at the end of this chapter. But you don't have to sit down with a cushion or spend an hour in a yoga studio to live more mindfully. You can integrate mindfulness into every activity in your daily life, from walking to cooking to doing your rehab exercises.

All you need to do is tune your focus in to the task at hand, paying close attention to every sensory detail—how things look, sound, smell, feel, and taste. Really focus on what you're doing. If your mind wanders—and it will—notice that and gently return it to the present moment. Cues—like Kirsten Cooper's beaded bracelet, or a mantra written on a sticky note or a piece of clothing—can help you remember. The process might feel a bit awkward at first, but the more you practice mindfulness in these small, everyday ways, the more likely it is that you'll be able to harness it in the most challenging situations you'll face during your recovery.

Success beyond question

American David Wise was the first-ever men's freeski halfpipe gold medalist at the 2014 Olympic Games in Sochi. In February 2018, he won gold again in PyeongChang. In between came the worst years of his life.

Some of the challenges Wise faced had nothing at all to do with his sport. His sister Christy, an Air Force pilot, lost her leg and nearly her life in a hit-and-run boating accident. His father-in-law died, and his wife Alexandra had postpartum depression after the birth of their second child, who then had a terrifying febrile seizure. On top of all this came injury—three concussions, chronic back pain, and a hard fall at the Mammoth Grand Prix in January 2016 that separated his left shoulder.

Wise had been used to winning every competition he entered, but in 2017, he didn't claim a single victory. Commentators and critics began predicting his retirement. Some of his sponsors, even those he'd had for years, broke their contracts with him.

But Wise also had the experience of purposefully handling setbacks. At the age of nineteen, he'd had his first ACL tear—and in what is truly an impressive cognitive feat for a teenager, he realized that the utter devastation he was feeling in the aftermath meant he was basing far too much of his identity on his athletic ability. He set out to rebalance his life, indulging his creativity and interests in writing and sport psychology. He practiced accepting what he couldn't change, adapting the way he responded, and acting to move forward. "Joy is a choice," he told us in an interview. "Happiness is a reaction to good circumstances, but joy is choosing to be content and happy no matter what happens to you."

Heading into 2018, Wise trained hard on skis, but also reinforced his mental preparation with mantras and visual reminders. Before each competition, he wrote a mantra in fabric pen on his left arm. One of his go-tos was "Embrace the opportunity"—a reminder to set aside performance anxiety and look at each run as a chance to excel, to show people the beauty and fearlessness of his sport as he spins through the air.

In Korea last year, he chose a new reminder: "You cannot fail." His seasons of struggle had taught him just how much was outside his control, he said. If he worked his hardest, performed his best, and still didn't win, he now knew he could honestly still count the day a success.

During the 2018 Olympic finals, success was far from guaranteed. Halfpipe scoring takes the best of three trips down the course, with flips and tricks judged on things like difficulty, variety, and height. In both of his first two runs, on the very first trick, he crashed, his skis popping off. "David Wise is running out of time," the announcer proclaimed as the skier stomped away in frustration.

Quickly, though, he accepted that he couldn't change the first two runs, and put them out of his mind. He stayed in the moment for his third run, which was flawless. Scores in the sport go up to 100. Judges awarded him a career best of 97.20—enough to edge out his teammate Alex Ferreira for gold.

Wise said that he knows his worth is not determined by any single competition, or even by a cumulation of them. Even so, after all he'd been through, that victory tasted even sweeter. At first, he was angry at those who had doubted him. Eventually, however, he realized that those emotions didn't serve him and he chose to feel gratitude instead.

The mental skills he'd practiced got him through yet another difficult period in April of 2019, when he broke his femur during an event in Austria. He documented the experience in a YouTube series called Overcoming, where he shared both the low moments and the attitude and techniques he used to rise above them. In fact, he began to see the injury as an opportunity to find his voice, to reach out to all types of athletes and share what he'd learned about resilience and mental strength with a wider audience.

Did you catch the rebound? Wise bounced when he stopped letting external circumstances dictate his emotions and instead chose joy. He bounced again when he turned anger at those who questioned him into gratitude for his injury experiences.

JUST THE FACTS

◆ Injury can make you feel entirely out of control.
◆ When you remain focused on the things you can't control, you amplify your negative emotions and experiences.

- If you rewind back to the past or fast forward to the future, you take your focus away from the present moment and what you need to do right now.
- You have more power than you realize, including possessing the ability to shift your emotional state.
- When you remind yourself of what's still within your control, you increase your feelings of confidence and motivation.
- Mindfulness—the ability to stay in or return to the present moment—is one of the most powerful mental skills you can have as an athlete, and as a human.
- Emotions are transitory. How you feel now is not how you will always feel.
- It's important to learn from the past and plan for the future—but your power to take action exists only in the present moment.

MENTAL SKILLS AND DRILLS

How can you bring yourself back to the present moment like Kirsten Cooper, learn without judgment like Amelia Boone, time-travel with intention and gratitude like Jennifer Nicely, set aside despair and failure to make room for the performance of your life, like David Wise? These exercises will allow you to recognize and move past what you can't control, focus on what you can change, and act in a way that propels you forward.

MENTAL DRILL: TIME-TRAVEL LOG

Gain awareness of the self-talk that keeps you rooted in the past or anxious about the future.

Mental Skills:
Level 1, Rookie: Focus
Level 2, All-Star: Self-Awareness
Level 3, Hall of Fame: Mindfulness

In the same way that a GPS watch tracks your route, you can keep tabs on the times when your energy and focus wander from the present moment back to the past or forward to the future. Use the template on the next page for your time-travel log. Commit to filling it out at least three days in a row. Choose a time when you know you're likely to have some negative thoughts about your injury.

For each thought, note down the date and time you had it, what self-talk you had in that moment, whether or not the thought was connected to the past or the future, what the situation was, and what emotions you felt. At the end of the three days, review your time-travel log and see if you can pick up on any themes. Simply making yourself aware of these trips is the first step in giving yourself the power to reduce their impact. From there, you can use drills like Feel and Focus and Energy Conservation—coming up on pages 89 and 90–91—to take control of them. Recreate the log below on a blank sheet of paper—or you can find a template in the workbook available to download from www.injuredathletesclub.com.

DATE/TIME	SELF-TALK	PAST OR FUTURE	SITUATION	MOOD

MENTAL DRILL: IN/OUT OF CONTROL

Pinpoint the factors you can change and those you can't influence.

Mental Skills:
Level 1, Rookie: Focus, Stress Management
Level 3, Hall of Fame: Discipline, Mindfulness

Reminding yourself of the things that are still within your control—even when you're injured—can feel empowering and keep you in the present moment. Create your own two lists of things that are in your control and things that are out of your control at this moment. Any time you are feeling frustrated or stuck, ask yourself if what you are contemplating is in or out of your control. If it's something that's out of your hands, how can you shift your focus to something that is within your power to influence?

IN CONTROL	OUT OF CONTROL
Doing my at-home exercises	How long it takes for my body to heal
Asking for support	What my teammates say to me

MENTAL DRILL: FEEL AND FOCUS

Identify how your emotions are affected by where your attention is focused.

Mental Skills:
Level 1, Rookie: Focus, Motivation
Level 2, All-Star: Attitude, Emotional Intelligence, Self-Awareness
Level 3, Hall of Fame: Mindfulness, Resilience

We never recommend running away from your feelings or denying your emotions. When you are feeling frustrated, angry, hurt, or sad, you want to lean into it rather than push it away. However, you also want to recognize that once you have leaned in and honored that feeling, it's OK to then choose to feel another way. The "Feel and Focus" drill below gives you a script to shift your focus and with it, your emotional state. Use it any time you need to pull yourself out of a negative mindset:

I am feeling _____ because I am focused on _____.

(Example: I am feeling hopeless because I am focused on the fact that I am not at practice.)

I want to feel _____, so I will focus on _____.

(Example: I want to feel optimistic, so I will focus on improving my skills.)

MENTAL DRILL: MINDFULNESS MEDITATION

Use meditation apps or simple exercises to calm your mind and accept what is.

Mental Skills:
Level 1, Rookie: Focus, Stress Management
Level 3, Hall of Fame: Mindfulness

Many people feel intimidated by the idea of meditating.

"I can't sit still that long."

"I can't make my mind be quiet."

"That sounds like torture."

Yet, for something as simple as sitting still, research has shown meditation to have wide-ranging benefits. Regular practice improves concentration, boosts the immune system, reduces stress, helps with sleep, and minimizes pain—all key for injured athletes. Traditional meditation is incredibly powerful, but there are many different ways you can practice mindfulness to strengthen your ability to calm your mind.

If you want to try seated meditation, start with five minutes; it's often easiest to do so at the same time every day (say, right after you wake up in the morning). Try creating your own meditation space—perhaps with a soft, comfortable cushion—that serves as a designated spot to sit and be still. Once you're there, take a few deep breaths and then close your eyes. Choose one thing on which to focus your mind, such as:

- your breath
- completing a body scan, in which you move your focus from head to toe and back again, noticing sensations and feelings
- repeating an injury mantra from Chapter 3, or a positive affirmation, such as one of those you'll develop in Chapter 8.

Your goal isn't to stop thinking—that actually isn't possible. Rather, you're aiming to simply to notice when your mind is wandering and bring it back to your point of focus, without judgment.

Some sessions will feel easier than others; don't expect to experience instant bliss every single time. However, consistency does pay off. Once you feel comfortable with five minutes, increase the timer by one minute; when you're comfortable with the extra minute, increase it by another minute, and so on. Another popular option is to start with guided meditation, using apps like Calm, Buddhify, or Headspace (which has packs specifically for sport performance and recovery).

MENTAL DRILL: ENERGY CONSERVATION

Visualize reining in your mental powers to focus on the present moment.

Mental Skills:
Level 1, Rookie: Focus, Stress Management
Level 2, All-Star: Visualization
Level 3, Hall of Fame: Mindfulness

When you find yourself feeling overwhelmed or scattered, or if you catch yourself time-traveling and need to bring yourself back to the present moment, turn to this drill. Start by making a mental list of everything on your mind right now. What are all the different problems, situations, or concerns occupying your mental space? What are you thinking about? *Who* are you thinking about?

Now imagine your energy as an entity, something that takes on form and shape—often, athletes will use a ray of light or a string. The precise image doesn't matter, just give it some sort of shape that extends from you and literally travels out to physically connect to places representing your thoughts. If you're thinking about what you need at the grocery store, imagine that beam of light extending all the way out to where you go shopping. Are you dwelling on an upcoming competition you'll miss or the one in the past in which you got hurt? Imagine that string stretching from you out to the venue. Take a few deep breaths while considering that image, noticing how it feels to have your energy extended so far. See if you can begin to physically feel that pull in your body. When you're ready, visualize slowly bringing that energy back towards you. See that ray, string, or other physical manifestation of your energy actually retracting. As it comes toward you, notice how you feel. Imagine that, as you slowly rein it in, you can detect a surge—the power of bringing 100% of your energy into the present moment.

MENTAL DRILL: RANDOM REMINDERS

Surprise your future self with motivational alerts.

Mental Skills:
Level 1, Rookie: Confidence, Motivation, Stress Management
Level 2, All-Star: Attitude
Level 3, Hall of Fame: Generosity, Resilience

Since we've been talking about time travel, you're going to send some inspirational messages to your future self. Set some "reminders" in your phone that will ping you with notes about how amazing you are. Think of messages that will tap into your strength and resilience as well as some that just make you laugh out loud:

- ◆ You got this.
- ◆ You're getting stronger every day.
- ◆ You ready? Who do you want to be today?
- ◆ Your torn ACL is super sexy.
- ◆ Who's the toughest injured athlete on the planet? This guy.

Choose any that resonate from this list and also create your own. They will hold more power when they are personally meaningful to you. Then choose random dates in the future and set reminders. Set some of them so far ahead that you forget you even put them in your phone. You'll be amazed at the timing of some of these when they pop up. If you have a teammate, friend, or trainer you trust enough to hand over your phone to, ask him or her to program a few for you. It's one great way to ask for support (you'll find many more in Chapter 6!).

MENTAL DRILL: WRITE IT OUT

Take pen to paper and use writing to move from frustration to acceptance.

Mental Skills:
Level 1, Rookie: Stress Management
Level 2, All-Star: Attitude, Emotional Intelligence
Level 3, Hall of Fame: Psychological Flexibility

Even if you lack the talent of Shakespeare, have terrible handwriting, and have never once kept a journal, you can still benefit tremendously from the power of working through your emotions on the page. For whatever reason, the act of writing can move you through emotions and toward acceptance. That's especially true if you're still feeling stuck in regret, wishing your injury had never happened. Carrying that psychological burden can weigh you down throughout your life and have an especially negative influence on your injury recovery.

For this mental drill you will:

1. Choose a time when you can commit to writing for four days in a row.
2. On each of those days, choose a time and place where you can have complete solitude and won't be interrupted.
3. Set a timer for twenty minutes.
4. As soon as you start the timer, start writing and don't stop until you hear the timer go off (it's OK if you go over time a little, but don't go over too much). Don't censor yourself. Don't question what you're writing. Don't question the direction you're heading in with your thoughts. Just write.
5. Do this FOUR DAYS IN A ROW.

If you commit to the exercise, you will be amazed at what comes from it. Even Carrie's most skeptical clients—those who claim to hate writing—have been awestruck by the emotional baggage they've been able to shed through the tips of their pens.

Note: The power in this mental drill lies in the act of writing. What you do with your written words after that is up to you. Some people read them right away, others set what they've written aside and read it a year (or several years) later. You might keep it and never read it again, or throw it in the trash or burn it as part of the ritual of letting go. Regardless of what you do with it, you've set down your load by writing, clearing up valuable mental space and releasing energy you can use to move toward recovery.

CHAPTER 5

CALM DOWN AND CHILL OUT

"You can find the positive in anything. I never really see anything as negative—I think half of the battle is mental."
—*Marathoner Jordan Hasay*

We often use the word "stress" to refer to the feeling of having too much to do and not enough time to do it. But the term has a more precise physiological meaning, especially for injured athletes. The kind of stress that is caused by injury results in the release of a cascade of hormones and nervous-system signals that impede healing, increase your risk of re-injury, and decrease your pain tolerance. Fortunately, however, you can prevent a potential stressor like injury from becoming a full-blown trigger of this physiological stress response by eliminating some stressors and managing your response to others. With practice, you can also monitor and tame one of the ultimate stressors for injured athletes—pain—while minimizing excess anxiety.

From tragedy to triumph

To say elite runner Jordan Hasay was facing pressure before the 2018 Boston Marathon would be a bit of an understatement. She was one of the few American women tipped to possibly win the race—and there hadn't been a female American win since 1985, six years before Hasay was even born. The year before, she'd run her first marathon in Boston, finishing third with a time of 2:25:53. That represented the fastest female US marathon debut by nearly three minutes.

In the weeks leading up to the race, Hasay had struggled with ankle and foot pain from plantar fasciitis and irritation of her posterior tibial tendon. Though past scans had been inconclusive, an MRI the day before the race showed a clear fracture line in her foot. That evening she dropped out, before even having the chance to battle the driving rains and 25mph headwinds that would make the 2018 Boston Marathon one for the record books. Desiree Linden, instead, became the first American woman to claim victory in more than three decades.

Though this was her first major injury, Hasay was no stranger to obstacles and setbacks. Five months before her first Boston Marathon in 2017, Hasay's mother, her best friend, had passed away suddenly. Hasay was devastated. To cope, she began journaling, writing letters to her mother that she wove through her training logs. She leaned on her support system, growing closer than ever to her coach, her dad, and her younger brother. During the race, she envisioned her mom running beside her.

So the next year, when faced with the prospect of not running for four weeks, Hasay felt confident she could weather the storm, and harnessed the same types of coping mechanisms she had used to handle her grief (use the Can You Cope? drill on page 114 to start building your own library of ways to cope). After allowing herself time to feel disappointment, she reframed her injury as an opportunity to grow. She returned to her journaling (do some writing exercises of your own in the Write It Out drill on pages 92–93). She noted flexibility as one of her weak areas, and started focusing on yoga to address it. She set mini-goals—new poses to master, thirty more seconds in headstand—and called her dad excitedly when she achieved them.

Hasay began running again in the summer, first with a mile, then with a few more. During her first speed workout, in June, she and her coach both noticed how much more fluid her stride seemed as a result of her time on the yoga mat. She hit a few more bumps—she was training to run the 2018 Chicago Marathon but had to withdraw a few weeks beforehand due to another fracture in the same foot. After another slow but steady return, she placed third again in the 2019 Boston Marathon. The flexibility, efficiency, and strength she's built, she believes, will serve her well as she looks toward the 2019 Chicago Marathon and the 2020 Olympic trials.

Did you catch the rebound? Hasay bounced when she coped by leaning on her support system and journaling. She bounced again when she celebrated each milestone of her recovery along the way.

SIDELINED AND STRESSED OUT

Stress affects all humans, athletes and non-athletes alike. In one way, injury counts as just another less-than-ideal experience. In reading this book, you might have noticed that many of the techniques we recommend for managing injuries could easily be applied to other stressful situations or obstacles you'll encounter in your life. In some ways, in fact, your body doesn't really differentiate between sources of stress, so similar tactics can help in a wide range of situations.

On the giant "Stressometer" scale, injury ranks quite highly in terms of emotional impact. First, there's the fact that you can't use your body the way you want to or participate in the sport that you enjoy (and that, maybe, earns you your livelihood). You're cut off from your social support system. You may even be questioning your entire athletic identity. In addition, physical activity acts as a release and an outlet for stress, but you might not be able to take quite as much advantage of it as you usually do. Add all that up and injury can feel incredibly overwhelming—your heart rate and breathing are probably starting to speed up just reading about its effects!

If that is indeed the case, sit with it for a minute, recognizing the real physical effect your thoughts are having on you. Then imagine you're looking at a fly through a magnifying glass—its shiny wings, spindly legs, and beady eyes appear terrifying! But if you put the glass down and step back, you can see that it's just an ordinary household pest. Think about whether you can consider your injury in the same way, even for a moment. When you think only about your current setbacks, as if through a magnifying glass, they appear larger than life. But if, instead, you can place them on a larger timeline of stressors in your life and your athletic career—all the losses and failures and injuries you've already endured, and will endure in the future—you can see it as difficult but manageable. You can and will get through it, and it's just another brief blip on a much longer timeline.

As you make this shift, you may notice your body feels different. Often your muscles relax a bit, and the pounding in your chest subsides. By noting those physical cues you've already begun to experience the tremendous power you have to control your stress response. (And that's just one of many stress-management strategies to come.)

As with so many other parts of the recovery process, the mind and body are intricately and inextricably connected in the stress response—what starts in your mind sweeps through your body. Psychological or physiological events can trigger the stress response—a phenomenon that, in turn, has both a psychological and a physiological impact. The way you manage stress can change your physiology and influence the progression of your healing, deep down at the cellular level. So, if injury is a stressor and stress can impede the healing process, what's an injured athlete to do?

THE PSYCHOBIOLOGY OF STRESS

The first step in defusing stress is to understand it. Of course, there are even more complex and fascinating biological processes taking place here than we have room to fit in this book—but even a basic understanding may help you grasp why this is so important to take seriously.

The experience of stress actually breaks down into two parts: the stressor and the stress response.

⬥ A *stressor* is a stimulus (usually an activity or event) that has the potential to trigger the stress response. Hitting traffic when you're already running late, fighting off a cold, being given an unexpected deadline on a project, getting injured—these are all examples of stressors. Stressors don't automatically become *stressful*, but all stressful situations begin with a stressor, or at least with the thought of one.

⬥ The *stress response* is your body's reply when you have assessed a stressor to be a threat, whether perceived or actual. You might have heard this called your fight-or-flight response. It's your body's defense system against potential danger.

We're evolutionarily designed to react quickly and subconsciously to threatening situations—that's what makes us able to dart away from a saber-toothed tiger or even react without thinking to score a game-winning point. In brief, the stress response begins when you gather sensory information about a potential danger. Your eyes and ears send data to an area of the brain called the amygdala, which quickly judges whether there's a true threat.

When your amygdala senses true trouble, it sends warning bells to another part of the brain, called the hypothalamus. You can think of the hypothalamus as the mission control center of your physiology—it's what activates both the accelerator (the sympathetic nervous system) and the brake (the parasympathetic nervous system) of your stress response system.

When you're under pressure, your hypothalamus hits the accelerator, sending signals to your pituitary and adrenal glands to produce stress hormones such as cortisol, norepinephrine, and epinephrine (aka adrenaline). These chemicals prepare your body for action. Your blood pressure rises, your breath and heart rate speed up, your muscles tense, and glucose rushes into your bloodstream. Even the airways in your lungs open wider, sending more oxygen to your brain and muscles. You're alert, awake, and ready to flee or attack—and all this occurs before you even have a conscious thought about what's happening.

Once the threat has passed, your hypothalamus hits the brakes, engaging the parasympathetic nervous system to slow everything down. You may have heard this called the "rest and digest" system. Blood returns to areas of your body, such as your gut, that weren't essential when you faced imminent danger. Your breath slows, and you start to relax.

In other words, the sympathetic system is speeding things up while the parasympathetic system is slowing things down. They're not always diametrically opposed—they work together to monitor the world around you and respond appropriately. Think of it in the same way as getting your shower to the perfect temperature by adjusting both the hot and the cold water. Together, these systems work in tandem to return you to homeostasis, or a state of equilibrium.

This immediate physiological reaction mobilizes efforts to respond to real threats ("Gather the troops, we're going to war!"). While this comes in handy in a true battlefield situation, the very same system can also kick into gear for a *perceived* threat ("Gather the troops, we're going to our first school dance!"). Things like traffic, deadlines, and discos aren't actual threats to your physical safety, but they can trigger your stress response if your brain decides they are a threat to your *psychological* safety.

What's worse is that unlike, say, staring down a saber-toothed tiger, these mental or emotional threats aren't always resolved swiftly. Chronic stress can throw the HPA axis—the complex network of the hypothalamus, pituitary gland, and adrenal glands—even further out of whack, making it more difficult for your parasympathetic nervous system to do its job of calming you down.

Let's go back to the list from Chapter 2 of unknowns that athletes typically face, as well as the dreaded "what-ifs" from Chapter 4:

◆ How long will my recovery take?
◆ Will I get my fitness back?
◆ When will I (or even will I) be able to train and compete again?
◆ Is there still going to be a spot for me on the team?
◆ Will I be the same athlete I was before my injury?
◆ If I do have to walk away from my sport, who will I then be?
◆ What if I don't make it back in time for playoffs?
◆ What if I don't come back as strong as I was before I was injured?
◆ What if the doctors can't fix me?
◆ What if my teammates don't trust me?
◆ What if I lose my starting spot?
◆ What if I get injured again?
◆ What if I can't come back at all?

Again, you're probably feeling stressed out just reading those. You can see how these unknowns and what-ifs, things that *might* happen, can quickly turn into perceived threats. It's another way our big, smart brains sometimes work against us. Most animals mobilize their stress response only with an immediate threat in front of them. We humans, however, can trigger our stress response simply by *thinking* about potential stressors. In these cases, triggering our physiological stress response does us far more harm than good.

"You're going to worry yourself sick" has a certain truth to it. Chronically triggering your stress response can be detrimental to your healing, your rehabilitation, and your likelihood of a successful return to sport. Research illuminates many detrimental physical effects of ongoing stress, including many that are particularly relevant to the injured athlete:

◆ Your tissues grow and repair more slowly
◆ Your immune system doesn't function as well
◆ Your sleep is disrupted
◆ You tire more quickly
◆ Your muscles don't get a chance to rebuild
◆ Your risk of re-injury rises.

These factors have a significant impact on your body's ability to heal and on your rate of recovery. All this means that managing stress isn't just some touchy-feely nonsense that only sensitive snowflakes need bother with—it's actually a critical component of your rehabilitation process.

What's more, absorbing and committing to this idea now can also prevent future injury. As an athlete, you might be used to hearing messages about toughening up, pushing harder, and not falling behind. However, the best athletes know that if you want to play hard, you have to recover harder. Research backs up this cultural shift—for example, a German study showed that professional soccer players who were highly stressed and unable to cope effectively were more likely to get hurt the next month.

Of course, we aren't explaining all of this to totally freak you out about feeling stress during your injury recovery. Adding a layer of stressing out about how much you're stressing out will do you no good. However, bringing awareness to the psychological and physiological processes underlying your stress response arms you with new information to counteract them. When you realize you are beginning to engage the stress response in the face of a *perceived* threat and not a real one, take a breath and see if you can reframe it. Think to yourself, "Ah yes, my body is doing what it is designed to do. But right now, triggering my stress response is causing more harm than good. So what do I want to do about it?"

FOUR KEY WAYS TO COPE

Of course, that's sometimes easier said than done. The good news is that you can build a mental toolkit of stress management resources, and we're going to help you assemble it. The more often you employ effective coping strategies, the more skilled you'll become at using them.

Back to the main question: If injury is a stressor and stress can impede the healing process, what's an injured athlete to do? First, know that your body follows your brain—so if your brain detects something stressful, your amygdala sounds the alarm to the hypothalamus, which then triggers the stress response in your body. However, not every stressor generates the same degree of response. When your brain evaluates each demand—each potential stressor—you consciously or subconsciously decide whether you are capable of meeting that demand. This assessment is based on your answers to three key questions:

◆ Am I confident in my ability to handle the situation?
◆ Have I successfully addressed this situation in the past?
◆ Do I have the support and resources necessary to meet this demand?

If your answers to these questions indicate you can handle the stressor in front of you, you take action to do so. If you don't, that's when the *stressor* becomes *stressful*. Employing coping strategies can shift the balance from feeling like you're overwhelmed to acknowledging that a situation is challenging, but feeling that you can manage it. Staying on the positive side of this equation will positively influence your ability to adhere to rehabilitation as well as your feelings of motivation and competence—all of which can get you back in the game more quickly.

There are four main coping styles: problem-focused coping, emotion-focused coping, avoidance coping, and support-seeking coping. Each encompasses several strategies and plays an important role in managing the stressors of injury recovery.

- *Problem-focused coping* directly addresses the challenge you're facing. Strategies include seeking out information, developing a skill, or setting specific goals. Problem-focused coping eradicates the stress by taking action on the things that are within your control—in other words, identifying the problem and then taking action to fix it.
- *Emotion-focused coping* focuses on the emotional response being triggered by the stress. Rather than act to change the stressor, these strategies lessen its impact. Examples include things like breathing and relaxation exercises, reframing the situation, and mindfulness and acceptance (for more on this, see Chapter 4). This may be the most appropriate coping style when many aspects of the stressor are out of your control, as can often be the case soon after an injury.
- *Avoidance coping* deals with the negative emotions of the situation by steering clear of the circumstances that bring them up. This can be done deliberately and strategically or out of caution or fear. Avoiding stressful situations is not necessarily a bad thing; in fact, it can be quite effective. However, if done over an extended period and in a manner that keeps you from moving forward, it's counterproductive.
- *Support-seeking coping* means looking to others to buffer the effects of stress. These strategies include asking for assistance, seeking feedback, and venting frustration. We will talk more extensively about seeking support in Chapter 6.

Back to the scenario of going to your first school dance. Here are ways you could use each coping style to address that particular stressor:

- Problem-focused coping: Take time to learn some sweet dance moves beforehand.

◆ Emotion-focused coping: Combat the physiological symptoms of the stress response by using some breathing exercises.
◆ Avoidance coping: Don't go to the dance.
◆ Support-seeking coping: Go with a group of friends so you have other people to dance with (and hide behind).

And here's how it might look in the case of a stressor common among injured athletes—testing out your injured body part with a new rehabilitation exercise:

◆ Problem-focused coping: Get more information by asking the trainer why they think your body is ready for this exercise.
◆ Emotion-focused coping: Visualize yourself successfully completing the exercise and remind yourself you're ready for this.
◆ Avoidance coping: Do a different exercise until you feel ready.
◆ Support-seeking coping: Talk to other athletes who have experienced your injury about how they knew they were ready to try a new exercise.

CHANNEL YOUR COPING

Now, you understand the different types of coping. Armed with this information, you can take a step back each time anxious sensations arise and you start to feel your stress response kick in. Instead of feeling overwhelmed, sit down and ask yourself:

◆ Which coping style am I using to address this problem?
◆ Is this the most effective style I could be using?
◆ What can I change to feel like I'm capable of meeting the demand in front of me?
◆ What strategies can I use to address the problem I am facing?
◆ What strategies can I use to address my emotional response?

Just thinking about the situation as a "problem" can help make a shift in your mindset. Thinking of it as "stress" can make it feel overwhelming and all-encompassing. But problems have answers, solutions; you can take steps to address them. By proactively using coping skills to manage the stressors you face, you are getting back in the driver's seat, taking an active role in your recovery rather than remaining a passive participant on the journey.

Let's take a look at how a real-life athlete has employed these coping styles to navigate his injury journey.

A complete coping toolkit

In college, Joshua Spokes worked to build the cycling team at the University of Maryland from a group of around five to one of the biggest teams in a conference. Spokes—yes, that's his real last name—twice qualified for USA Cycling Collegiate Road National Championships. After school, he moved to Spain and continued to ride and compete.

Throughout his career, Spokes has incurred both traumatic injuries—broken bones and concussions in crashes—and overuse injuries, including Achilles tendinitis, patellar tendinitis, and an ongoing hip issue possibly related to a torn labrum. Here's how he's coped with setbacks.

Avoidance coping: One of Spokes' first major crashes came during his senior year of college, not long before his final exams. He went to the university health center and got notes allowing him to defer his final exams and projects until he'd recovered from the effects of his concussion—alleviating the stress of pushing toward his academic goals when he wasn't prepared.

Problem-focused coping: In navigating his hip injury, Spokes sought physical therapy and studied up on some of the underlying biomechanics by reading *Athletic Body in Balance* by Gray Cook. The book contains self-tests and exercises that have allowed Spokes to work on—and track—things like his flexibility and mobility.

Support-seeking coping: Spokes surrounds himself with other expats in Spain—those who don't cycle. He's also reconnected by phone and text with his family. And he's connected with other injured athletes, both by joining The Injured Athletes Club on Facebook and by creating videos that he then posts online to share what he's learned about the injury-recovery process.

Emotion-focused coping: Each day he's off the bike, Spokes fires up the Headspace app. The guided meditations provided there allow him to stay in the moment and cope with the emotions that bubble up when he isn't able to ride as a way to help manage his stress and problems.

To keep all his coping mechanisms on track, Spokes uses a paper journal to track his habits, marking off the days he successfully sticks to his plans. By focusing on positive habits when injured, he's better able to maintain them when he's healthy and riding again.

THE BIG-WHAMMY STRESSOR: PAIN

In one way, pain is a physical and inevitable part of the injury process. It's a signal from your body to your brain that something's not right—a tendon's torn, a bone's broken, a ligament's sprained. But as the stories from injured athletes in this book illuminate—and as you may have noticed in your own experience—the severity of an injury doesn't always correlate with how much it hurts.

Pain can also guide you during your rehab and recovery, but it's not always interpreted then in the same way as it is, say, immediately after surgery, when pain is something to be alleviated or avoided. In rehab and recovery—during therapy exercises, for example—discomfort must be endured or even encouraged. The type of pain you're experiencing (where it's occurring, and whether it's sudden and sharp or dull and aching) also plays a role in how you might want to respond to it. And all of this is complicated by the fact that there's no objective test or measure of pain. Only you can truly experience and explain the degree and quality of the pain you're experiencing.

All this means that pain merits an extra degree of attention in the rebound process. Here, in brief, is how pain occurs during the injury experience:

1. Infliction: Damage occurs to one of your body's tissues, triggering pain receptors.
2. Nociception: Information about that damage travels from those receptors through your nervous system to your brain.
3. Perception: Your brain makes sense of the signals it's receiving, influencing how much pain you actually feel.
4. Reaction: Higher-level brain processes determine how important the pain is and what to do about it, influencing both your tolerance of pain and your behaviors in response to it.

Though it often starts with physical damage, pain isn't always a reliable indicator of injury severity. In part, that's because of the complexity of our physiology. Sometimes injuries occur in areas where pain receptors aren't present. In other cases, scrambled nerve signals exacerbate minor pain, cause it to linger longer than the damage that triggered it, or else eliminate the sensation of pain even when our tissues are severely compromised.

The other reason pain and tissue damage don't completely align is because your psychology and your emotions have a significant impact on nearly every part of the process. The way pain signals travel, your perception of pain, and your assessment of what it means and how to handle it are based on many factors beyond the physical, including:

◆ whether the pain was anticipated or unexpected
◆ how you've dealt with pain in the past
◆ how much information you have about what's causing the pain (Remember ultrarunner and obstacle course racer Amelia Boone from Chapter 4? She had thirteen MRIs to investigate pain the year after her second stress fracture—they all came back clean and, magically, her pain disappeared.)
◆ the stage you're at in your recovery
◆ emotions such as anger, anxiety, and depression
◆ your level of trust in your medical team, especially your physical therapist/athletic trainer
◆ fears of re-injury; pain that was once perceived as a normal part of training or competing can be seen differently in light of these anxieties
◆ cultural messages about how athletes "should" respond to pain, including the fact that suffering is sometimes seen as a sign of mental toughness
◆ how worried you are about your coaches' and teammates' opinions about your pain
◆ your confidence in your ability to handle the pain, including whether you have a plan to manage and respond to it.

Your emotional reaction to your pain can prevent you from staying present and getting feedback about the qualities of the pain. Consider these two scenarios:

◆ You feel pain as you start doing rehab and immediately feel anger: you're angry with yourself, with the people involved, with the fact that you can't compete.
◆ You just got cleared to return to practice and experience some pain on your first day back, and you feel fear: fear that you're not really ready, fear that you won't be the same, fear of re-injury.

In both of these cases, your emotions cloud your ability to learn from your pain and to then take appropriate action.

The good news is that as an injured athlete, you can do a lot to influence your perceptions and reaction to pain. That way, you can treat it as a physical sensation that often provides valuable information about your injury and recovery. To make this mindset shift:

◆ Understand your pain. Get as much clarification as you can on "normal" versus "problematic" pain. Your medical team plays a key role here. At each visit, ask what pain you might experience and what you should do about it (for example, stop an activity, seek medical attention, or simply find ways to reduce or manage discomfort). Between visits, you can use the pain log (on pages 112–113) to record your pain and then discuss it with the medical team on your next visit. Talking with other athletes who have similar injuries and doing online research can help too—though it's best combined with personalized advice. Reassess regularly as your injury recovery progresses.

◆ Soothe pain physically. Pain medications help in some circumstances, such as post-surgery (see box about this on page 108). Your medical team can advise on other external ways to ease pain that are normal and non-threatening, including use of ice or heat, massage or other bodywork, hydrotherapy, and laser or electrical stimulation.

◆ Reduce pain emotionally. When you know that the pain you are experiencing is not a signal to stop, but a discomfort that comes when you are asking your body to push toward recovery, there are two different strategies you can use: **dissociative** or **associative** strategies. **Dissociative** strategies seek to distract you from the pain you're feeling by drawing your attention somewhere else. Listening to music, talking to other people, thinking about your grocery list, or replaying your best performance in your mind are all examples of dissociative strategies. **Associative** strategies do the opposite, tuning you into the pain. You don't fight the pain or try and hide from it, but instead breathe into it and stay psychologically present. This keeps you in tune with what is happening in your body so that you'll know when it's OK to push and when you need to back off.

You might not be able to take away the physical aspect of your pain, but you can manage your emotional experience through relaxation and self-talk strategies aimed at lessening the intensity of your pain. The next time you are faced with doing a rehab exercise that hurts, or when you're suffering from getting back into high-intensity efforts after time off, try preparing for the pain by giving yourself a pep talk. Think or say out loud: "I'm strong enough to do this. My body can handle the effort." Then breathe deeply through the discomfort.

A NOTE ABOUT PAIN MEDICATIONS

Your medical team may recommend over-the-counter (OTC) or prescription medications to help manage pain while your injury heals. In addition to making you more comfortable, some medications can reduce inflammation and increase your mobility so that you can more easily do appropriate rehab exercises. Ask your doctor, therapist, or trainer about OTC drugs like naproxen, ibuprofen, or acetaminophen/paracetamol.

For severe pain—such as immediately after a traumatic injury or surgery—your doctor or surgeon may prescribe opioids or other pain medications. These drugs offer powerful relief—but carry significant risks, including the potential for dependence or addiction. A 2017 consensus statement from the International Olympic Committee advises doctors to prescribe these drugs to athletes at the lowest dose possible for the shortest time possible, preferably no longer than five days. They also should consider an athlete's history with substance abuse and establish clear goals for pain management and improved function.

Because medications like opioids can influence your thinking and memory, they may influence your psychological response to injury and recovery; emotions may be muted while you're taking them and then unpredictable when you stop. It's important to recognize these effects and work closely with your medical team to manage your medications and safely transition off them. Talk with your doctor if your pain doesn't improve within a few days of your injury or surgery. And for anyone experiencing problems with opioid dependence, the Substance Abuse and Mental Health Services Administration's National Helpline is available at 1-800-662-HELP (4357) in the United States. U.K residents can call Talk to Frank on 0300 123 6600.

Harnessing healing energy

Adam Whiting was an aspiring musician who found yoga in his mid-twenties as a way to manage his anxiety, and eventually earned his teacher certification. He joined a prominent studio in Australia and began teaching other teachers, leading workshops, and headlining yoga festivals.

As his career as an international yoga instructor blossomed, so too did a nagging case of chronic back pain. He bounced around to a variety of different providers and received an equally variable array of diagnoses, from sacroiliac (SI) joint instability to a problem with his lumbar ligaments. Whenever the pain worsened, he'd modify his practice and seek acupuncture, dry needling, or massage. Those kept the pain under control until Christmas of 2016, when, during a yoga class in Australia, Whiting demonstrated a handstand in class and felt a strange tweak. The next day he was flying back home to America to teach at workshops. He felt OK on the first day, Friday; after the second, he could barely stand up; and on the Sunday, he taught from a chair.

For a while, he continued seeking non-invasive treatment from chiropractors, even as his pain grew so severe he could barely walk. Fearful of becoming dependent on pain medications, he used only over-the-counter ibuprofen. He combined that with yoga nidra, a guided-meditation technique employed to manage pain, anxiety, and depression.

One morning, Whiting tried to stand up to let his dogs out and couldn't—his left leg was numb from the knee down. He tried to drive to the doctor himself and, in searing pain, pulled over and called a cab. Fortunately, he was able to see a neurosurgeon quickly. His disc had essentially extruded, wrapping around his spinal nerves. Surgery was the best option, he was told. Whiting scheduled the procedure for four days later.

Fortunately for Whiting, the operation was a near-instant success; as soon as he woke up, the pain was dramatically decreased. Still, recovering from surgery wasn't exactly easy. He timed one of his first walks and laughed to see he had covered one kilometer in forty-seven minutes.

As he prepared to return to the mat, he'd lie in bed and envision moving through an entire practice. "The main reason why we practice yoga asana, the movement, is to move energy around the body … you don't need to move the body to move the energy," he said. "I would finish a practice and I would lay in *savasana* [corpse pose], which ultimately I was in the entire time, and I felt completely renewed."

When he could resume more of his regular activities, he felt profound gratitude for every movement. Two weeks after surgery, he was allowed to drive again. He thought back to the day when the pain was so great he couldn't operate his own vehicle. "A routine and reflexive process that I had never given a second thought to was now a gift," he said.

Did you catch the rebound? Whiting bounced when he used yoga nidra to manage his pain. He bounced again when he visualized himself completing yoga poses from his bed, and when he channeled gratitude for his regained function.

JUST THE FACTS

- Stress results in a cascade of hormones and nervous-system signals that impede healing, increase your risk of re-injury, and decrease your pain tolerance.
- For an athlete, injury is a serious stressor, one that packs a significant emotional impact.
- Chronically triggering your stress response can be detrimental to your healing, rehabilitation, and likelihood of a successful return to sport.
- You can trigger your stress response simply by thinking about potential stressors.
- Coping strategies shift the balance of stress from feeling overwhelmed to acknowledging that a situation is challenging, but that you can manage it.
- Pain is a signal from your body to your brain that something's not right and an important guide during your rehab and recovery.
- Our emotions and past experience play a key role in how we perceive pain and in what we do about it.
- You can manage your emotional experience through relaxation and self-talk strategies to lessen the intensity of your pain.

MENTAL SKILLS AND DRILLS

How can you harness your obstacles and turn them into fuel like Jordan Hasay, use coping skills like Joshua Spokes, tame pain and mentally redirect your energy like Adam Whiting? The following exercises will help you reduce sources of stress and anxiety when this is possible, and calm your body's response to them when it isn't.

MENTAL DRILL: R&R

Learn breathing exercises and other physical ways to defuse the stress response.

Mental Skills:
Level 1, Rookie: Stress Management
Level 2, All-Star: Visualization
Level 3, Hall of Fame: Discipline, Mindfulness

When it comes to stress management, you can either relax the brain in order to relax the body or relax the body in order to relax the brain. The first are called *mind-to-muscle* techniques, the second *muscle-to-mind*. The following mental drills are muscle-to-mind techniques—physical actions that help relax the body in order to relax the mind. Choose from the options below next time you need to bring your stress level down a couple of notches.

Sigh of relief. Stress, tension, and anxiety can disrupt your normal breathing pattern, causing you to hold your breath or breathe shallowly. Sighing is your body's natural and automatic response to help restore a normal breathing pattern. Take in a deep breath, then let out an audible sigh.

Chew therapy. Research has shown that chewing gum can help reduce anxiety and lower levels of cortisol. For a bonus mood booster, reach for the gum you used to chew when you were a kid. It's hard to be upset when you're blowing bubbles with a mouthful of Big League Chew or Hubba Bubba.

Rhythmic breathing. The power of this breathing exercise is in the pause. Inhale through your nose to a count of four, hold your breath for a count of four, and then exhale through your mouth for a count of four. Try it for a few breaths; even raise your shoulders just a bit as you inhale, and then feel them drop as you exhale. As you improve, try increasing to a count of five or six.

Roses and candles. Combine breathing and visualization for a one-two punch against stress. Close your eyes and deeply inhale through your nose as you imagine smelling a beautiful, fragrant rose. Actually see the rose in your mind as you inhale. As you exhale, blow forcefully out of your mouth as if you're blowing out a candle on a birthday cake.

Calming countdown. Start with a few deep breaths first, and then begin. As you exhale, count down from five to one. With each decreasing number, tell yourself you're becoming progressively more relaxed, releasing any tension from your body and mind. Physically and mentally feel yourself letting go until you hit the number one and the tension is gone.

Serenity on cue. Again, start with a few deep breaths. When you're ready, add a cue word to your inhale and exhale. Your cue words are triggers for how you want to feel in this moment. For example, as you inhale, think "Confidence"; as you exhale, think "Calm." Choose from the following list of words or use your own:

Confidence/Calm
Strength/Courage
Power/Persevere
Relaxed/Ready
Excited/Determined

Relax, bit by bit. Practice passive progressive relaxation by releasing tension from each muscle group, one by one. Start with your feet and legs and move your way up your body. Inhale and bring your attention to a new body part. With your exhale, imagine allowing that muscle group to relax. Take two breaths in each area. Pay attention to how each muscle group feels as it loosens (you might even visualize stress flowing out of the body). You can also find guided progressive relaxation exercises on many popular meditation apps.

MENTAL DRILL: PAIN LOG

Objectively track and describe your pain.

Mental Skills:
Level 1, Rookie: Focus
Level 2, All-Star: Communication, Self-Awareness

Some pain is "normal" and OK to push through, while other types of discomfort mean you should pull back before you worsen your injury. The challenge? Telling the difference. Creating a pain log can help you gain a deeper understanding and awareness of the pain you're experiencing. Recreate the log below on a blank sheet of paper—or you can find a template in the workbook available to download from www.injuredathletesclub.com. Fill it out each time you feel pain, and share it with your treatment team. Together, you can figure out the best way to handle each type of ache.

DATE	ACTIVITY	
Pain intensity (circle one):		
Mild	Moderate	Severe
Pain rating on a scale of 1 to 10 (1 is little to no pain, 10 is intolerable)		
My pain rating is:		
When did pain occur? (circle one):		
Before	During	After
Quality of pain (circle all that apply):		
Sharp	Aching	Throbbing
Stabbing	Burning	Shooting
Tender	Numb	Stinging
Other notes:		

MENTAL DRILL: ANXIETY PYRAMID

Rank events that make you feel nervous and visualize successfully overcoming your anxiety one step at a time.

Mental Skills:
Level 1, Rookie: Confidence, Goal-Setting, Stress Management
Level 2, All-Star: Self-Awareness
Level 3, Hall of Fame: Visualization

Anxiety is one of the many emotions that occur during your injury journey—one that gets a pretty bad rap. Our natural urge is to reduce or eliminate it. But anxiety is an important emotion, provided you lean into it and listen to it.

For this mental drill, create a list of eight to ten things related to your injury and your recovery that produce anxiety. Include everything from items that produce just a tiny bit of discomfort all the way to the ones at the very top of the pyramid that make you so scared they're hard to even think about. Then, rank each item in order. Put those that produce the least amount of anxiety at the bottom or base of your pyramid, and those that fill you with fear and dread at the top.

As you proceed through rehab and recovery, aim to tackle each item in order. Start by visualizing yourself successfully accomplishing one item at the bottom of your pyramid—then go out and do it. Once you feel calm and confident at that step, you can move up to the next. Don't fret about what's at the top of the

113

pyramid, just focus on taking one step at a time. As you begin to see success, you'll gain motivation and confidence to continue toward the peak.

For example: sketch a pyramid based on the anxiety around getting back on your bike after a crash. At the bottom of the pyramid might be "Looking at your bike." Then: "Bringing your bike into your living room," followed by "Sitting on your bike," "Riding your bike indoors on the trainer," "Taking a short ride outdoors on a protected course," "Going longer on an open road," and at the top, "Riding in the same spot where you had your crash." You can find an example in the workbook at www.injuredathletesclub.com.

MENTAL DRILL: CAN YOU COPE?

Match potential stressors with effective coping techniques.

Mental Skills:
Level 1, Rookie: Goal-Setting, Stress Management
Level 2, All-Star: Self-Awareness
Level 3, Hall of Fame: Resilience

On page 102 we discussed the four different coping styles: problem-focused, emotion-focused, avoidance, and support-seeking. Brainstorm a list of all the stressors you are experiencing right now. They can be both injury and non-injury related—all stressors impact your injury recovery. For each stressor, choose a coping style you feel would best manage it, then come up with at least one strategy within that style. Be sure to refer to the "Grab Your Goals" mental drill in Chapter 3 to turn these strategies into effective goals.

STRESSOR	STYLE	STRATEGY
Doctor's appointments	Emotion-focused	Deep breathing before the visit
Uncertainty about when I'll return to training	Problem-focused	Ask for information from my trainers and medical team
Media is replaying the video of my injury	Avoidance-focused	Turn off the TV and use caution on social media until the attention has subsided
Trouble getting around due to limited mobility	Support-seeking	Ask for a ride or a hand carrying things

MENTAL DRILL: STRESS BUSTERS

Brainstorm ways to banish stress, from simple mood-lifters to major lifestyle changes.

Mental Skills:
Level 1, Rookie: Focus, Stress Management
Level 2, All-Star: Self-Awareness
Level 3, Hall of Fame: Generosity, Resilience

You can't eliminate all stressors in your life, but relieving the tension caused by the ones you can't eliminate helps restore balance. Create two lists, one titled "Stress Balancers" and the other titled "Stress Relievers." Stress balancers are things that alleviate and balance out some of the stress you are under—physical ways to reduce the stress response. Stress relievers are things that bring you a sense of relaxation or joy. See the examples below, and come up with your own. Once you have your two lists, set a goal each week for how you will manage your stress in such a way as to help your injury recovery.

STRESS BALANCERS	STRESS RELIEVERS
Getting eight hours of sleep	Creating a mood-boosting playlist
Booking a massage	Watching a funny movie
Seeking support	Reading
Meditating	Journaling

CHAPTER 6

RALLY YOUR CREW

"If I'm constantly around positive people who are pushing me to be better, I'm going to become better. If I'm around people who are negative and don't believe in the things I'm doing, I can't expect to elevate my performance."
—*CrossFit athlete Scott Panchik*

Injury can leave you feeling weak and alone. But the truth is, you have tremendous power to steer your recovery, and that power is amplified when you have a crew to assist you. All injured athletes can benefit from a variety of different types of support throughout the recovery process. The challenge comes in cultivating a network to provide that support, especially at a time when physical limitations may isolate you from your usual team or community. This starts with recognizing what you need—and then being brave enough to ask for it.

The team approach

For Scott Panchik, CrossFit has always been intimately linked with family and community—and recovery. His father first introduced him to the sport when Panchik was still a running back at the University of Mount Union. During his junior year, Panchik tore his ACL, his MCL, and his meniscus playing football. His two younger brothers were seriously hurt in a hiking accident. The father and three sons used CrossFit as a type of rehab and therapy.

When Panchik moved to Ohio for a teaching job after graduation, he sought out the same sense of camaraderie at a CrossFit gym in his new city. He began to realize he had real potential as a CrossFit athlete, and wondered if he could even reach the sport's three-day televized world championship, the CrossFit Games. He did so in his very first year trying—and placed fourth in the 2012 CrossFit Games.

Panchik met his wife through CrossFit; their first date was at the gym. Eventually, he dedicated himself to the sport wholeheartedly. His brothers moved to Ohio to join him in training and they opened their own gym, CrossFit Mentality.

Like all athletes pushing themselves to the limit, Panchik continued to face injury. During his second year at the Games, he caught a snatch wrong and tore his bicep, an injury requiring surgery. Though some doctors told him he'd likely never have the same mobility in his shoulder again, he found others who supported his ability to recover completely (prepare to communicate clearly with your healthcare providers using the Here's What's Up, Doc drill on pages 134–135). In consultation with them, Panchik thought about how he'd train an older person with limited function if they showed up at his gym, and proceeded that way.

As well as giving him an appropriate physical challenge, the athletes and coaches around him provided a psychological boost. When he stayed home on the couch, his thoughts turned dark. But when he surrounded himself with others aspiring to achieve goals, he felt motivated, willing to put in the work he needed to recover.

With that attitude, Panchik came back from that injury, and continued to make the CrossFit Games each year. He headed into the 2015 competition with a case of plantar fasciitis, an overuse injury involving inflammation and pain in the tough tissue running along the bottom of the foot. During the first event of the Games—which involved running on the beach, then swimming—Panchik stepped out of the water onto a sand dune and felt a pop. That band of tissue along the bottom of his foot, his plantar fascia, had partially ruptured.

Of course, he didn't know that at the time. All Panchik knew was that he hurt. The medical staff at the Games provided immediate support, helping him manage the pain. Still, he wasn't sure if he could make it through all three days of competition. He called his wife—at the time his fiancée—who immediately came to be with him. With her support he harnessed all the mental strength he'd acquired through years of workouts, injury, and recovery and finished the competition, placing sixth.

Note: We're not suggesting you must keep pushing through a painful injury to be considered strong or successful. Panchik made that risk-and-benefit calculation for himself, and told us: "I spent, like, 360 days out of the year training for those five days. People would kill for the opportunity to just even run out onto the floor. So in my mind I felt like it was worth everything." What's key, we think, is that even a super-tough CrossFitter like him didn't do any of it alone.

Did you catch the rebound? Panchik bounced when he joined his father and brothers for active rehabilitation at CrossFit. He bounced again each time he left the comfort of his couch to put himself in an environment where he'd feel motivated to recover.

SIDELINED AND SHUT OUT

The people you train and compete with are often more than just your teammates—they also become your friends. During certain parts of the season you probably spend more time with them than with anyone else. So when you're injured, it's more than your athletic identity that takes a hit—often, you also lose a big part of your community.

Everyone benefits from social support. In 1938, researchers recruited 724 participants to carry out the longest study ever conducted on health and happiness. The Harvard Study of Adult Development has spanned the length of eighty years. The original researchers chose a range of males, from Harvard college graduates from the most advantaged families to inner-city Boston kids from the most disadvantaged families. Over those eighty years, they peered into every facet of the participants' lives to see what they could understand about happiness and health.

From eighty years of research on the 724 men, there was one very clear and undeniable outcome: *the men who had good relationships and strong social connections were happier, healthier, and lived longer.* The message was clear—having good, close relationships matters. Time spent with others has a buffering effect on the stressors of life.

Now, these particular results involved only one type of participant—Caucasian men. But many other studies have similarly shown that social support positively affects the health and wellness of a whole range of other populations, and, specifically, injured athletes. In one Ohio State University study, injured athletes who reported satisfaction with support from their athletic trainers were less likely to have symptoms of depression or anxiety when returning to play. In another, involving 224 injured collegiate athletes, those who had social support reported greater overall well-being.

Why is this so? As we discussed in Chapter 5, your psychological response to stress can be either beneficial or detrimental to your mental and physical health. Social support bolsters your defenses against the stress of being injured, enabling you to cope better. And then there's the fact that support can also provide you with resources that speed and ease your recovery, from information about your diagnosis and prognosis to help wrapping a sprained ankle or getting around when you're less mobile.

Social support comes in two forms: perceived and received.

◆ *Perceived social support* is your belief that, should you choose to seek it out, support will be readily available to you. You might not need any kind of help at this exact moment, but you feel you have a good network of resources and access to assistance should you require it.

◆ *Received social support* is the actual support that is being provided to you. You've reached out for help—and your call has been answered.

Interestingly, sometimes perceived support is actually more important to an injured athlete than received support—but we'll get to that in a minute. For now, it's important to understand that having both of these types of support—perceived and received—allows you to experience your injured status as less stressful and believe in your ability to power through and come out the other side.

Injury is an emotional roller coaster. When you have people there to buckle up next to you for all the ups and downs, it's not quite as terrifying a ride. It's time to rally your crew.

THE FOUR TYPES OF SUPPORT

First, the nuts and bolts of support. From the onset of your injury to the moment of full recovery, you'll come across quite a few situations that require outside input or assistance. There are four different types of support you will need throughout your rehab: emotional, tangible, motivational, and informational. Each one is essential in your quest to rebuild yourself into a stronger, healthier athlete.

TYPE OF SUPPORT	ATHLETE EXAMPLES
Emotional support: *Boosting your psychological well-being by:* ◆ getting in touch with you to check that you're OK ◆ allowing you to vent your frustrations ◆ listening without passing judgment or giving advice ◆ expressing empathy, care, and compassion ◆ acknowledging how much it sucks to be injured	Minneapolis runner Jessie Benson and her husband Dustin had spent three years—and thousands of dollars—planning a trip to Antarctica to run a marathon. Three weeks before they were due to depart, Benson slipped on the ice and broke her tibia and fibula in multiple places. From excitedly counting down the days until the race on her blog, *The Right Fits*, she now had to turn her timeline from five weeks to the race to fifty-six, in the hope of getting to go the following year. "I got into a bit of a dark and depressed state for a couple of days and I was really bummed about it," she said. Talking to other athletes and reading their comments on her blog played a key role in lifting her out.
Tangible support: *Providing discernible acts of assistance, such as:* ◆ driving you around ◆ carrying things like books, bags, and medical supplies ◆ making or bringing you food and running other errands ◆ helping with scheduling ◆ getting equipment out to the field for modified workouts with your team	In the weeks after surgery, Jessie Benson couldn't do much. Her husband went out in an ice storm to buy her a shower stool, then wrapped her wounded leg in a duct-taped trash bag before she got under the spray in order to keep it dry. He and her friends took turns driving her to her Crank Cycle class, an upper-body workout that was one of the few ways she could elevate her heart rate; as there was no elevator at the gym, they escorted her up the stairs while carrying the scooter she was using to get around. Another friend, a personal trainer, designed specific workout routines incorporating Benson's limitations.

TYPE OF SUPPORT	ATHLETE EXAMPLES
Motivational support: *Inspiring confidence and creating momentum by:* ◆ offering task-specific encouragement ◆ checking in on your recovery progress ◆ celebrating milestones with you ◆ reassuring you and believing in you ◆ being a rehab or goal buddy	Swimmer Greg Wells broke his neck in a freak surfing accident, but was determined to compete again. At one point during his comeback—when he was swimming again but far below his prior fitness level—he was slowing down at the end of a lap when a teammate slammed him into a wall during a flip turn, then told him he'd better keep going. At first Wells was shocked: "I had a broken neck and he just kicked me as hard as he could!" But looking back, he remembers it as a turning point. "No one in my group ever let me stop again. My teammates were so positive, so encouraging, so supportive," he said. "It wasn't just me. Everyone else was invested in the fact that I was trying to come back from this, and that made all the difference in the world."
Informational support: *Providing wise counsel and essential knowledge by, for example:* ◆ offering advice from the perspective of an athlete who has experienced the same injury ◆ explaining different options for treatment ◆ providing helpful advice and suggestions ◆ breaking down what pain is normal and what pain you should pay attention to ◆ designing appropriate rehabilitation exercises to do and suggesting goals to set during recovery	When British duathlete and cyclist Nikalas Cook fell and fractured his patella while running, he knew exactly who to turn to: his friend Phil Burt, the physiotherapist for Team Sky and the Great Britain Cycling Team. Burt tried to persuade Cook's surgical team not to put the leg in a cast, due to potential muscle mass loss. His efforts weren't successful, but he did get Cook transferred to a top surgeon to oversee his recovery. Burt then designed a complete rehab program, which had to be flexible to account for unintended obstacles, such as the pinning and wiring technique used to hold his bones in place during the healing process. While all this was happening, Cook's work colleague mentioned that his brother had also broken his kneecap, and put the two athletes in touch. "It was so good to talk to someone who'd suffered the same injury, especially as he was back to full racing fitness. He'd really pushed with his rehab and it gave me a real boost to do the same," Cook said.

Thinking about these four types of support can get you off to a good start in planning out what help you'll need (check the Build Your Team exercise on page 133 for specifics on starting this process). Of course, surprises will come along, but doing your best to predict your needs in advance will go a long way toward relieving your stress right now—and will assist your recovery later on.

ARE YOU READY TO BE SUPPORTED?

Despite the fact that their social support network has a huge impact on an athlete's recovery, many athletes steer clear of seeking out and asking for the support they need. Can you identify yourself in any of the following three categories?

REASONS PEOPLE DON'T ASK FOR HELP	IS THIS YOU?
They don't want to be perceived as incompetent.	You are fearful of asking a "stupid" question or of being judged. You don't want to look incompetent or feel embarrassed, so you'd rather just try to figure it out on your own. You may even feel like you should somehow inherently know the answer or be able to do it without help, so you avoid asking your coaches and healthcare providers questions, even if the answers might be important for your recovery.
They don't want to be perceived as needy.	You don't want to inconvenience people or be a burden. You avoid asking for help at all costs, and when you do ask, you tend to immediately backpedal into saying that you don't really need it. You may also fear rejection. Emotionally, it is easier to not need help than it is to be denied help.
They don't want to be perceived as weak.	You believe that asking for help is a sign of weakness and that showing weakness makes you vulnerable. You think that it says something negative about your character and who you are as a person. To you, it means you have failed because you have put the control into someone else's hands and think that asking for help might come at a cost. It might threaten your position on the team, or it might threaten your view of yourself.

You can see how these beliefs would lead someone to make the choice to not seek out support.

But what if you flipped it? This idea taps into the research of Carol Dweck, author of the book *Mindset*. Dweck wanted to understand why some people rise up in the face of a challenge while others shrink away. The simple but profound idea she discovered in her research is that it all came down to a person's mindset—and specifically, whether they have a *growth mindset* or a *fixed mindset*.

When you have a growth mindset, you believe that traits like your intelligence and talent can be developed over time—and that success is possible through your efforts and strategies, and with assistance from others. When you have a fixed mindset, you believe that your qualities are set in stone and can't be changed, and that success is only achieved through those innate talents. Asking for support, therefore, is akin to failure.

The people who are the most successful at facing challenges have a growth mindset. They don't see asking for help as a sign of incompetence, neediness, or weakness. They view it as the opposite. Seeking out resources, asking for help, and requesting support are assets essential to their success.

When you play out the idea of not seeking assistance in other scenarios you can recognize its absurdity. Not asking for help during your injury recovery would be like deciding to pick up a manual or watch a YouTube video to figure out how to replace your own carburetor, even though you've never worked on a car before, because you don't want to be viewed as incompetent by hiring a car mechanic. Or like learning how to fly a plane before your next trip because you don't want to "be a burden" to the pilot with twenty-plus years of commercial flight experience. Or like tearing your ACL and deciding to go ahead and perform the reconstructive surgery yourself. Somehow, you *should* be able to do that on your own; you wouldn't want to look weak by letting someone else do it for you.

It's easy to recognize these situations as ridiculous. Of course we need help! The same holds true when we're dealing with injury. With that in mind, let's look at some core beliefs about asking for support through a growth mindset.

I WILL ASK FOR HELP BECAUSE:	THIS IS ME:
I want to be perceived as engaged and informed.	Asking questions shows you are intelligent and competent enough to seek to understand what's happening to your body. You are an active member of your healthcare team—and if you have accurate and complete information, you, your coaches, and your healthcare providers can work together to make your recovery faster and more successful.
The people around me want to support me—and they care about my well-being as much as I care about theirs.	You are not a burden, and you deserve health and well-being just as much as anyone else. Although you may encounter a time when a specific person can't or won't provide the support you need, generally speaking, the people around you want to know how to help you and will welcome guidance on how to do so. The connections you make or deepen during times of struggle are often among the most lasting and rewarding, and propel everyone involved to higher levels of achievement.
I want to prove that I am strong.	Even if a few misinformed people see asking for help as a sign of weakness, the most successful athletes know they cannot reach their peak performance at any stage without the support of others. The very fact that it is hard to ask for help means that it takes a tremendous amount of courage to actually do so.

DO YOU HAVE A SAFETY NET?

It's not too hard to understand how an appropriate rehab plan, a ride to the doctor's office, or even a sympathetic friend to console you aids in your recovery from injury. But remember we mentioned that *perceived* support—the belief that help is available should you need it, even if you don't need it right now— also plays a critical role in your recovery? In fact, as we also hinted at, research shows that *perceived* support actually has a *greater* stress-buffering impact than *received* support.

That seems counterintuitive at first, but when you think about it a little bit, it starts to make sense. If you feel like you're trying to manage and recover from your injury all on your own, you're probably going to feel high levels of stress all the time. Even if you're not in pain or don't have a question at that precise moment, you're living on the edge, feeling like you're only one step away from falling off the cliff with no one to rescue you. On the other hand, if you know you'll have support when you need it, you'll be more confident in your ability to handle difficult situations even when they do arise.

As well as our natural independence or stubbornness, our previous experiences are among the things that hold us back from adopting a growth mindset toward injury and accessing perceived support. We know we warned you against time-traveling too much in Chapter 4, but this is an instance where it's beneficial to answer a few questions about what's happened in the past so that you can learn from them. Ask yourself:

- What kind of messages have you received in the past about asking for help?
- Was independence valued more than collaboration, or vice versa?
- How have people responded to you when you've reached out for help?
- How do you view people who have reached out to you for help?
- Do you trust that support will be there for you when you need it?

We recognize that many athletes' answers to these questions will provide evidence against the desirability of relying on perceived support. Maybe you've asked a teammate for help and she shot you down. Perhaps your doctor or coach reacted poorly when you posed a question about your rehab. It could even be the case that you've looked down on someone who's come to you for support in the past, and you don't want to create that reaction in others.

But here's where we're going to ask you to take a little bit of a leap of faith and start to work on changing your beliefs about support in spite of some conflicting evidence. What's extra compelling about changing to a growth mindset surrounding support—recognizing you need help, and making the decision to request and accept it—is that it actually increases your ability to take advantage of the incredibly powerful resource that support represents.

Here's how: Your brain will selectively pay attention to the aspects of your interactions and experiences that meet your preconceived notions. The underlying beliefs you have about asking for help inevitably influence your perception, your behavior, the way you communicate, and the choices you make. If you show up to therapy (or skip it altogether) convinced you don't really need help from your physical therapist or trainer to improve, how is that session going to go in comparison with the time you arrive eagerly looking forward to the guidance of an experienced pro? If you fail to reach out to your teammates because you think they don't want to see you while you're hurt, they may get the message that you don't want to see *them*, and stop including you, further limiting your social interactions.

The way you think about what it means to ask for help can actually influence how likely you are to receive that help—and therefore, whether you're able to benefit from the valuable resource that support represents. Sometimes it starts with just a small action, a request that seems simple but begins to restore your faith in the power of support. Even if you've been burned in the past, we hope you'll consider reaching out again. Ultimately, you're the person who will benefit.

WHEN SUPPORT FALLS SHORT

As you think through your past experiences, there are a few other things to consider that might allow you to let go of any resentment or doubt about the times your crew has let you down. The reason it might seem as though the people around you aren't supporting you may be down to one of a number of possible mismatches:

- **Timing mismatch.** The support you need in a given moment might not be the actual type of support you are being offered. You might get emotional support from a friend when what you need is a kick in the butt, or vice versa. Or your doctor may start to drop some informational support on you when you're feeling angry and overwhelmed and need to hear that it's all going to be OK. Your negative reactions to these mismatches can be particularly confusing, even to you, because you recognize that someone is trying to help you but you wind up feeling worse.
- **Knowledge/skill mismatch.** Your recovery team and healthcare providers often want to support you emotionally, yet feel unqualified to do so. (There's no class yet on how to properly talk to injured athletes in medical or physical therapy school—though if we had our way, there would be!) And sometimes family and friends attempt to provide informational support, despite the fact that they have no idea what they're talking about. People often

support you in the way they would want to be supported or in the only way they know how, but that may not match your preference or current needs.

◆ **Communication mismatch.** Many misfires with communication can happen throughout your recovery. Doctors don't always think before they speak. Teammates and friends often say things that are unintentionally hurtful. You might not have expressed your needs clearly. And depending on your frame of mind, you may make inaccurate assumptions about the meaning behind someone's words.

Just understanding these mismatches can alleviate some of their sting. Here are a few more ways to prevent them, or to address them when they do occur:

◆ Build a multi-person team. No one human alone can fulfill all your needs as an injured athlete. The more hands there are on deck, the more likely it'll be that there's someone there to step up when you really need them, in the exact way you need.

◆ Match the team member to the task. You wouldn't hire a car mechanic to fly your plane or ask an orthopedic surgeon to fix your car. Similarly, relying on doctors for emotional support—or on less knowledgeable friends for informational support—might not be the best way to proceed.

◆ Practice compassion. Recognize people's strengths and weaknesses and be realistic about what kind of support you can expect on the basis of what they are willing or able to provide. You don't want to judge someone for what they can't offer. Instead, recognize what you need and accept that that person may not be best suited to meet that need.

The Communication Cheat Sheet exercise on pages 137–138 can help you ask for what you need clearly, and in so doing, reduce the risk of all three mismatches occurring. And the Found in Translation drill on pages 135–136 can help you reframe interactions that seem negative to you at the time they happen.

Knowing about these mismatches exposes these two key myths that lead to increased aggravation and frustration for injured athletes:

◆ Everyone in my life should know exactly what type of support I need and be able to provide it at the exact moment I need it.

◆ If people aren't supporting me, it means that they don't care about me and what I'm going through.

Wouldn't it be nice if that first myth were actually true? But it's clearly not, and neither is the second. It might help you to think about reversing the roles—it's obvious that you are not a bad person if you don't recognize that another injured athlete needs support, or if you give them a different type of support from what they are seeking at that moment. And during times when you aren't able to support someone, it doesn't necessarily mean that you don't care about them and their well-being. The same is true of the way people are around *you*—sometimes they just need more direction to know how to respond or behave. But if you give them the chance and they don't rise to the occasion, that's when you might want to re-evaluate the relationship or at least take a little break from it until you're both in a better place.

Note that you might find there are people in your life who are the opposite of supportive—who continually bring you down with their negativity. If it's possible, consider not spending time with people who leave you feeling upset or drained. When that's not possible—if they're your coaches, teammates, or family members, for instance—try using exercises like the "Found in Translation" drill on pages 135–136 or go through the Communication Cheat Sheet on pages 137–138 to manage your response to them.

BUILDING THE BEST MEDICAL TEAM

Trust in your healthcare team ranks highly on the list of factors that are important to your recovery. "It's critical—it's the cornerstone of everything that unfolds," says physical therapist Stephania Bell, a spokesperson for the American Physical Therapy Association and ESPN's injury analyst. So, choosing a quality team is key.

Your best outcomes will likely come from seeking out physicians who specialize in their sport or injury—someone who treats football players wouldn't necessarily be your go-to for a running-related overuse injury, advises Philip Skiba D.O., director of sports medicine at Advocate Medical Group in Chicago and also a trainer and coach who's worked with elite endurance athletes, including marathon world record holder Eliud Kipchoge. At your first visit, have a conversation about yourself and your injury. "If they're not willing to take that kind of time with you, you need a different doctor," says Skiba.

Ask questions like:

- How many times have you treated this particular injury?
- How many times have you treated athletes like me?
- What have their outcomes been?

Though cost might be a factor if you have to go through a medical insurance provider—and you might also be dealing with input from coaches, agents, and sponsors—good doctors never mind if you seek a second opinion regarding how to treat your injury. In fact, they expect it, especially if you're facing surgery or another major procedure. In many pro leagues, as Bell points out, second and even third opinions are written into collective-bargaining agreements.

Again, if your doctor doesn't welcome this, you should probably consider changing doctors, says Skiba. Quality healthcare providers should not only be open to you seeking another opinion, they may even connect and collaborate with other physicians as a means of finding the most informed and well-considered path forward for you, the athlete. (Note that this is different from shopping around simply to find a doctor who will give you only the answers you're looking for, whether that's a conservative approach or cutting-edge treatment, a faster or a slower return to your sport.)

Ideally, this coordinated team support should continue once you begin rehab. "I think the best relationships are the ones where everyone on the team is very communicative and collaborative," Bell says. "If there's not good collaboration within that team, then they start thinking: 'Which one do I trust?' That can affect the overall quality of care."

If you don't feel your team is collaborating or you have frustrations with your physician or surgeon, consider asking your physical therapist or athletic trainer—the person you see most—to intervene on your behalf. And if it's that person you're feeling frustrated with or unsupported by, it's also within your rights to seek out another option. "At the end of the day, I always say [athletes] need to advocate for themselves. If they're not feeling like they're in a good situation, then they need to be free to seek out another appointment or another alternative," says Bell.

Turning sorrow into strength

Ashlee Groover can clearly remember times she received the support she needed—and times she didn't. She'd had surgery for a torn hamstring, an injury that occurred not long after she moved across the country from San Diego to Pittsburgh to play softball for Robert Morris University.

Her dad was able to fly out for the days immediately following the procedure. After he left, Groover—who uses words like "hard-headed" and "independent" to describe herself—had to learn to ask for help with everything from carrying her books to class to daily hygiene. She'd bought a shower stool, but couldn't reach the shampoo and body wash, something she couldn't do without pulling her injured hamstring. Not only did she need assistance getting into the stall, someone had to sit in the bathroom the whole time, handing her bottles.

Groover lived in a suite with nine teammates, so there was usually someone to lend a hand. But one night everyone seemed occupied when it came time for her to clean up. She asked the person she thought she could rely on for assistance—and got a brisk "Aren't you OK to shower for yourself finally?" in return.

Now, it's possible that her teammate was purely being cruel. But as we've discussed, there are other potential explanations. There may have been a timing or communication mismatch—this teammate, who'd helped before, could have felt overwhelmed by her own study and practice schedule (learn how to give others the benefit of the doubt with the Found in Translation drill on pages 135–136). Undoubtedly, she didn't express her situation as kindly as she could have. Regardless of her intention, though, Groover felt devastated and decided to make her way into the stall herself, slipping and struggling as she did so. She sat in the streaming water for forty-five minutes, sobbing.

For a long while afterward, she felt even more reluctant to reach out. Her coaches didn't help the situation, rarely asking how she was doing. But eventually, she learned that continuing to ask for assistance was essential not only for her physical recovery, but for her psychological well-being, too. As she returned from her injury—and dealt with a nasty breakup at around the same time—she sought support at the school's counseling center.

Empowered by her experience, she returned to the team a stronger person. When she was injured in her senior year with a torn knee ligament that benched her again, she sought out a mentorship role with younger athletes. And she changed her entire major and career path to sport psychology, vowing to make it easier for other athletes to access the type of help she'd received. Now, she's at Springfield College doing graduate work in athletic counseling and working as the head counselor at the school's Sport Injury Rehabilitation Clinic.

Did you catch the rebound? Groover bounced when she recognized that she couldn't handle her stresses on her own and sought professional help from the counselor. She bounced again—big time—when she redirected her entire career, aiming to ensure that future generations of athletes have access to the support they need.

JUST THE FACTS

◆ You have tremendous power to steer your recovery; that power is amplified when you have a crew to assist you.

◆ Support has a significant buffering effect on stress, and lowering stress is critical for your recovery.

◆ To succeed in your rebound, you have to know what types of support you need—and then go ask for that support.

◆ The belief that you'll have support when you need it makes you more confident in your ability to handle difficult situations.

◆ Your ability to ask for and accept assistance from others is essential to your success.

◆ People aren't always great communicators. That doesn't mean they don't care.

◆ Matching the support crew member to the task makes it easier to get the type of help you need.

◆ Trust in your healthcare team is critical to your rehab.

MENTAL SKILLS AND DRILLS

How can you build a supportive team like Scott Panchik and Jessie Benson did, ensure you have appropriate medical care like Nikalas Cook did, even overcome negative experiences with seeking support, like Ashlee Groover did? With these exercises, you'll learn to identify your needs and who might address them, reframe negative interactions so they don't set back your progress, and speed and enhance your recovery by taking advantage of the incredible power of gratitude and support.

MENTAL DRILL: BUILD YOUR TEAM

Identify the people in your life who can provide each type of support.

Mental Skills
Level 1, Rookie: Confidence, Goal-Setting, Motivation, Stress Management
Level 2, All-Star: Communication, Self-Awareness
Level 3, Hall of Fame: Generosity

Injury may make you feel lost and alone—but in fact, you are the captain of your injury team. It's time to choose your players. Start this process by answering the following:

- What do you feel is the most important factor for you to have a successful recovery?
- Are there any questions you still have about your injury?
- What's your biggest concern regarding your injury recovery?
- Do you feel that you are facing any barriers to getting the resources you need for a successful recovery?

Take a look at the following needs and place them in the four categories described below: emotional, tangible, informational, and motivational. Then identify the people who would be able to provide you with that type of support. There's a page in the workbook, which you can download from www.injuredathletesclub.com, to create your own chart.

SUPPORT	EXAMPLE	RESOURCES
Emotional support	Someone to commiserate with you	1. Teammate who's been through an injury 2. Sister/brother/friend
Tangible support	A ride home after surgery	1. Roommate/partner
Informational support	A rehab plan	1. Athletic trainer 2. Surgeon
Motivational support	A cheerleader to celebrate milestones with you	1. Partner/friend 2. Athletic trainer/physical therapist

MENTAL DRILL: JOIN THE CLUB

Connect with your virtual tribe in The Injured Athletes Club on Facebook.

Mental Skills
Level 1, Rookie: Focus
Level 2, All-Star: Attitude
Level 3, Hall of Fame: Discipline, Psychological Flexibility, Resilience

Not only does being injured take you away from your teammates physically, it also sets up a psychological barrier. After all, even the people you feel closest to when you're healthy and performing well might not "get" you in the same way when you're injured. Fortunately, however, there *are* people who understand: other injured athletes. Find a new tribe in groups like The Injured Athletes Club (IAC) on Facebook. The IAC motto is: "We're sorry you're here but we're glad you're with us." It's a place to give high-fives, get group hugs, and share resources to help pave a smoother path on your road to recovery and beyond. Head over to www.facebook.com/groups/TheInjuredAthletesClub to join and share your journey with others in the same situation as you. You can also listen to The Injured Athletes Club podcast, where athletes and others in the field share their insights and lessons. You'll find links to all these resources at www.injuredathletesclub.com.

MENTAL DRILL: HERE'S WHAT'S UP, DOC

Build a toolkit for your healthcare appointments.

Mental Skills
Level 2, All-Star: Attitude, Communication, Self-Awareness
Level 3, Hall of Fame: Discipline, Generosity

Your doctor may know more than you about physiology and surgery—but you're a critical member of your treatment team too, and it's important for your questions to be answered and your voice heard. Preparing for each medical visit ensures that this will happen. Run through the following checklist each time you have a medical visit:

⬧ **List your questions.** If you don't go to the doctor's office with an agenda, you're going to be subject to theirs—and then you might leave feeling like your needs haven't been met. Use the sample questions

below to prepare your own in advance. Don't be afraid of the answers—
you need that information to alleviate your fears and know what your
next step is. If you have a long list, consider asking for an extra ten
minutes when you book your appointment, so that no one feels rushed.

◆ **Capture the responses**. Take a notebook or even a voice recorder with
you (but check first if it's OK to use it; some offices have policies against
recording, and it's always a good idea to get permission first). If you get
into a highly emotional situation during your appointment, when you
walk out of the office you won't remember one thing that was said to you.

◆ **Enlist back-up.** Consider bringing someone from your support
team with you as an advocate and a second pair of ears. You might
shut down when you hear something unexpected, or you might have
selective hearing and listen for what you *want* to hear, so your friend
or family member can be there to catch the things you missed.

Sample questions

◆ In your experience, how long does it take athletes with this type of
injury to return to their sport?

◆ What type and level of pain is normal at this point, and when should
I be concerned?

◆ Are there any other red flags that should prompt me to call you or
another healthcare provider?

◆ What activities can I do, and which should I avoid?

MENTAL DRILL: FOUND IN TRANSLATION

*Examine and defuse counterproductive assumptions during
interactions with others.*

Mental Skills
Level 1, Rookie: Focus
Level 2, All-Star: Attitude, Communication, Emotional Intelligence
Level 3, Hall of Fame: Discipline, Generosity, Psychological Flexibility

No doubt about it—some people are just jerks. But we've found you can get
a lot farther in life—and in injury recovery—when you at least begin by
giving people around you the benefit of the doubt. People aren't always great
communicators, and when someone else is in distress, they can get even more
flustered and easily say the wrong thing.

Plus, when you're coping with something like an injury, your own emotions can cloud your judgment. You can easily interpret someone else's statements and intentions in a more hurtful light than was intended. For instance, you might be in a place in your recovery when you just don't want to deal with a barrage of questions about what's happening and when you think you'll be back. Even though people ask out of concern and because they want to connect with you, when you're feeling emotional about your recovery, their words can push you over the edge.

This includes your medical team. At times they forget that they are not just talking to a body part, they are talking to a person—an athlete with hopes and dreams. They might not realize that if they start the conversation with, "Well, things aren't looking so good" instead of saying, "How are you feeling today?" you're liable to fear your world is crashing down around you.

For this mental drill, you're going to do a little editing of your interactions. Sometimes you have to translate people's words to get to what they really meant (or what would've been more helpful to say). Consider the following examples, and, on a separate piece of paper or the workbook available from www. injuredathletesclub.com, write down interactions you've had that felt hurtful to you, along with a different interpretation of each one. The more you practice this drill, the more generous you'll be in your interpretations—and the less words will sting you. Plus, you'll likely be more thoughtful about what *you* say to friends in tough spots, too.

Your doctor said: "Well, things aren't looking so good."	Your doctor meant: "I'm reviewing where you are right now and trying to figure out what we need to do for your progress."	Your doctor should have said: "Hello, great to see you! How are you feeling today?"
Your teammate said: "Jeez—I wish I could take that much time off from training. Ha ha."	Your teammate meant: "I feel awkward, like I don't know what to say."	Your teammate should have said: "I'm really sorry you can't be out here with us. I've been thinking a lot about you."
Your coach said: "Buck up."	Your coach meant: "I have a lot on my plate, but you're still on my mind."	Your coach should have said: "It's OK to feel overwhelmed. I know you're strong enough to handle this."
Your trainer/ therapist said: "I can't believe you've slacked on these exercises."	Your trainer/therapist meant: "I'm concerned about your recovery and worried that missing out on rehab is going to slow your progress."	Your trainer/therapist should have said: "It can be really hard to stick to a program. Let's talk about what's holding you back and find ways to make this work for you."

MENTAL DRILL: COMMUNICATION CHEAT SHEET

*Fill in the blanks for simple, straightforward ways to ask for help
or shut down critics.*

Mental Skills:
Level 2, All-Star: Communication, Self-Awareness
Level 3, Hall of Fame: Discipline, Generosity, Psychological Flexibility

The previous exercise focused on others' words—now, let's consider your side of the conversation. Putting some thought into how you'll respond to comments that come across as cruel or thoughtless not only removes some of their sting, it also prevents you from lashing out without thinking in reply. While responding sarcastically or angrily may feel good in the moment—and some people probably deserve it—your mood's likely to sink even lower afterward, especially if it turns out you misinterpreted what was said. Plotting out in advance how you'll ask for the help you need also makes those interactions go more smoothly.

Try out the following tactics, and pay attention to how they work for you—feel free to modify slightly if you find other words that feel more natural for you. And as you go through your recovery, keep an ear out for other effective ways of phrasing responses to sticky situations or requests (either things you say that work well, or things that you hear others saying). Make note of them to add to your own arsenal.

Projection
For people who tell you how you must be feeling, saying things like, "You must be so upset", or "Surely you're relieved to take a break?"
Instead of saying:
"Thanks for the heads-up on my own emotions, you jerk."
try:
"I appreciate your concern, but actually I'm feeling _____"
or "I can see why you might think that, but actually _____"

Disappearing Act
When you run into someone for the first time and you think they may have been avoiding you.
Instead of saying:
"Thanks a lot for *finally* showing up."
try:
"Hey! It's been a while. It's great to see you."

or "I actually thought you might be avoiding me. I know sometimes it can be hard to see someone when you're not sure what to say."

Storytelling
For people who respond to your situation by telling you a story about themselves or someone else—sometimes one that has an unhappy ending.
Instead of saying:
"Really? Why on earth would you tell me that right now?"
or "OK, I guess we're talking about YOU now."
try:
"I know you're trying to connect with me, but hearing that story makes me feel _____."
or "Wow, thanks for sharing. Do you think it's going to rain tonight?"
Note: Choosing the first option—or something like it—provides a powerful opportunity to educate those around you. But you don't have to advocate for yourself in that way every single time, you can also choose just to let the comments roll off you and move on.

Switcheroo
When someone asks about your injury and you just don't want to talk about it that day.
Instead of saying:
"Why can't you ask me about something else? I'm not just my injury."
try:
"Yeah, it's a big bummer, but I'm moving on. How are you doing? Tell me what's new with you?"
or "I'd certainly prefer not to be injured; I have good days and bad days. But I'd actually love to talk about something else."

I need you
When you need to ask someone for support.
Instead of saying:
"Why can't you just do this one simple thing for me?"
try:
"One of the things I value about you is _____ and one of the things I really need support with is _____."
or "I could really use some help with _____. Is this something you could help me with?"

MENTAL DRILL: GIVE THANKS

Express your gratitude to your support team through words and actions.

Mental Skills
Level 1, Rookie: Stress Management
Level 2, All-Star: Attitude, Communication
Level 3, Hall of Fame: Generosity

Think about the last time someone genuinely thanked you for something out of the blue or let you know how much of an impact you had on them. Think about how good that made you feel. Wouldn't it be wonderful to pass that feeling along to others? It's time to give thanks to your support team, to make them feel as good as they have made you feel by giving you their support. Showing gratitude to people can improve your relationships, which can also help with future communication. And guess what: Research shows that giving thanks makes the giver happier too! Since a big part of your injury recovery task is reducing stress and promoting positive feelings, this mental drill is a win–win.

What are some specific ways you can show gratitude to your support team? Who do you feel have been some of your biggest supporters? Who has helped you the most during this time? Think about people who helped you even in small ways. Send a thank-you card, take them out for coffee, throw a thank-you party. As you give thanks, tap into that feeling of gratitude.

CHAPTER 7

FEED THE (INJURED) ATHLETE

"The mind heals the body. There is no other way around this."
—Professional boulderer Bernd Zangerl

Thoughts have tremendous power to steer our recovery in a positive direction—
or to derail it completely. As you'll find out in this chapter, we all have a little
athlete on one shoulder and a monster on the other, each thriving on a diet of our
thoughts and beliefs. Every day, we make choices about which one to nourish.
When you're injured, the fear, doubt, and negativity that come along with
getting hurt can act like Miracle-Gro for your monster, naturally strengthening
it. Fortunately, you can regain control of this equation during the injury and
recovery process, and empower your inner athlete as your muscles, joints, and
bones repair and rebuild.

A vision of restoration

Austrian climber Bernd Zangerl was climbing in Cresciano, Switzerland, in 2015, when he fell. His tumble didn't seem that bad at the time. But a few days later, his neck stiffened and his head pounded. He woke up one morning with bloodshot eyes, and headed to the hospital. There, doctors did an MRI and told him he was lucky he wasn't paralyzed. He'd cracked one vertebra and badly injured another, damaging ligaments that surrounded nerves in his arms. Soon, he couldn't feel his thumb and index finger, a result of swelling around the damaged tissue. Hours later, his arm and shoulder muscles began to vibrate—a sign, he later realized, that his brain had stopped sending signals their way.

Doctors suggested surgery, but couldn't promise success. Zangerl declined. His shoulder and arm began to atrophy, to the point where he couldn't even lift a frying pan with his right hand. He saw specialist after specialist, some of the best in Europe. Many told him he'd have to give up on climbing altogether. But in his heart, he couldn't let go— something told him that even the smartest neurologists in the world didn't completely understand how nerves repair and rebuild.

Meanwhile, with his livelihood uncertain, Zangerl felt himself slipping into depression, losing his motivation to even get out of bed in the morning. Aware of the way his emotions would affect the physiological aspects of healing, he aimed to structure his days in ways that would lift his mood. In his calender, he would block time for yoga, reading, and spending time in nature. (Use the Stress Busters drill on page 115 to craft your own uplifting strategy.)

With his dreams of returning to climbing slipping away, Zangerl decided to take a break from doctors and gyms. From August to October of 2016, he went to the Himalayas, his happy place, by himself. While there, he began to meditate specifically on his injured body, focusing his energy on the muscles essential for climbing. Doctors had given him an electrostimulation machine to jump-start impulses between his brain and his shoulders and arms. Zangerl now attempted, through sheer concentration, to recreate that sensation of electricity traveling from mind to muscle. (The Healing Visions drill on page 73 shows you how to apply this powerful type of technique to your injury.)

His muscles felt warm—could it be working? Soon, he was able to climb easy boulders. When he hit a plateau, he decided to give the physical part of training a rest so his nerves could fully heal and to focus only on the mental. He began and ended each day with meditation, and continued his yoga practice, intensifying his sessions and studyding the mind in depth with his teacher, Roland Wäschle.

In February 2017, he passed a bouldering area on his way home from visiting a friend; on a whim, he put on his climbing shoes and laid down a crash pad. Soon, he realized he'd passed a difficult sequence he hadn't been able to send ("sending" is climber lingo for successfully ascending) years before, when uninjured. "In that came so much happiness and energy because in this moment I was sure I'm going to make it. Now I know it's just a question of training," he said.

By April 2017, Zangerl was climbing more intensely than he ever had. He now continues to meditate for an hour each morning and each night, not only focusing on activating his muscles but also picturing himself making successful ascents. And those doctors? "They came back to me and asked, 'What did you do? We can learn from you,'" he said.

Did you catch the rebound? Zangerl bounced when he purposefully planned his days in ways that would keep negative thoughts at bay. He bounced again when he began using visualization to foster healing, and when he rested to allow his nerves to regrow.

MEET YOUR BIGGEST CRITIC: YOU

During your injury process, you've likely encountered at least one person who criticized you, doubted you, or brought down your mood—whether it was a coach who made you feel unworthy, a fan who questioned your abilities, a doctor who discouraged you, a friend or family member who just didn't get it ... or all of the above. You probably recognized, quickly, the negativity they brought to your recovery process, even if you didn't always know what to do about it.

What you might not realize at first is that your own self-talk—the inner dialogue and constant chatter running through your head—plays just as big a role as the words of others, if not a bigger one. If you're constantly berating yourself, questioning your intentions, or doubting your abilities, you may subconsciously undermine your own goals of rehabbing successfully and returning to your sport swiftly. Meanwhile, if you're identifying your strengths, highlighting signs of progress, and eagerly anticipating your return, you'll find it much easier to sustain your confidence and your motivation to persist.

Carrie has long explained it this way: Each one of us has a little monster sitting on one shoulder and a little athlete sitting on the other. They each have goals they're trying to accomplish, with lots of ideas, opinions, and thoughts on how to get there. Your inner athlete believes in your ability, has confidence and courage, and is willing to take risks and dream big dreams. Meanwhile, your inner monster is fearful and full of doubt, is consumed with negativity and dismissive, and makes you feel like an imposter.

Your athlete and your monster are vying for your attention, and you are the one who decides which will get it. Whichever one you choose to feed—whichever one gets your attention the most—is the one that will grow stronger. For some, it feels like the monster is much louder and more vocal than the athlete. Injury often widens the gap further; the doubts and frustrations that come along with being sidelined are pure monster fuel. But don't despair: Feeding the athlete is a skill. You can get better at it—you may just need some practice.

You might be tempted to blow this off as self-help or pop-psych blather. After all, concepts of "optimism" and "positive self-talk" have been generalized to mean that if you just think happy thoughts you will be happy all the time and if you aren't happy, it's your own darn fault. This line of thinking makes Carrie want to turn into a monster herself, as it's just not true at all.

What *is* true is this: certain attitudes and mindsets can elicit unwanted and unnecessary stress; we have some ability to influence our emotional experience; and those thoughts and emotions have an influence over our behavior.

In short, self-talk has a real and measurable impact on your rehab, recovery, and ability to rebound. We typically tend to move toward things that make us feel good and away from things that make us feel bad. When you are feeling confident and hopeful, you're more likely to move *toward* recovery, taking the steps you need to get back out on the court, field, or course. When you're feeling fear and doubt, you are more likely to move *away* from those things because you are uncertain of the outcome. Your self-talk processes and directs your focus to influence how you act, feel, and perform.

THE MONSTER–ATHLETE BALANCE

We don't necessarily want to completely banish the monster. Buried beneath its snarls and growls, the monster voice might call your attention to something you've been neglecting, the "what-ifs" that you can prepare for once they've been voiced. Think about your monster and your athlete as buddies, teammates; they have to find a way to work together toward a common goal. Often, they truly do have the same goal—such as avoiding re-injury—though they often have very different ideas about how to get there. Let them have conversations with each other. In doing so, they can bring you back to homeostasis just like your sympathetic and parasympathetic nervous systems do. Here's an example of how this might play out:

	MONSTER	ATHLETE
Thoughts	"I'm afraid. I don't know if I should do this. I don't know if I'm ready for this."	"It's normal to feel that fear of re-injury. But I've been working hard and my body is getting stronger every day."
Emotions	Fear, doubt.	Nervousness tempered by determination and confidence.
Actions	Skip physical therapy appointments.	Work with athletic trainer on exercises to prevent re-injury.

Now, these are both valid strategies to avoid re-injury. However, one is driven by your desire and one is driven by your anxiety. In a case like this, imagine your inner athlete listening to your monster profess its fears and then countering them, rather than buying into them. You might actually imagine your athlete saying: "I hear your fears and concerns, little monster. I know what you're trying to do—protect me by sabotaging me—but I got this." Recognize that your monster is often fiercely guarding the gate of your ego, running or fighting to protect it at all costs. Your athlete needs to learn how to be the bigger voice, taming the monster so it doesn't grow huge and take over.

Fortunately, your inner athlete can thrive on a relatively varied diet. You can choose to feed the athlete in three key ways: with body language, with thoughts, and with imagery.

BODY LANGUAGE

Try out this little experiment: put yourself in the physical posture of defeat. Your head is down, your shoulders are slumped over, you're kicking the ground. Hold this posture and say to yourself, "I am strong. I can do this." Now shake that off and put yourself in the pose of someone who's standing confident and determined. Your head is up and you're looking ahead; your shoulders are back and chest is up; your feet are firmly planted forward. Hold this position and say again, "I am strong. I can do this." Notice a difference?

Your body language plays an important role in your emotional landscape. The next time you feel hesitant or anxious, notice your body language in that moment. Then take a breath and see if you can shift to reflect a position of greater confidence. Often, this physical repositioning jump-starts the shift in your mind. Your facial expressions play a role in this as well. Experiment with keeping a relaxed face rather than grimacing through a rehabilitation exercise or practice drill to see the difference in how you feel.

THOUGHTS

Your thoughts direct your focus. Again, we're not advising you to bury all negative thoughts or think only happy ones when you don't actually feel that way. Right now, we're not even talking about reframing the event to try and change how you feel about it. All emotions—including negative emotions—are fleeting. And in the same way a Snapchat disappears after you read it, acknowledging and calling attention to these negative emotions robs them of their power.

If you are about to do a rehabilitation exercise for the first time and find yourself feeling apprehensive, simply pause to recognize that emotion. If you can, verbalize it: "I'm feeling anxious." You may immediately feel calmer, relieved. Remember back to Chapter 5, where we learned about how your amygdala processes stress? You're much more likely to provoke your stress response when faced with something unknown or unexpected. When you label an emotion, you recognize what you're dealing with, calming your mind instead of being consumed by uncertainty and the feeling the emotion produces.

You can also shift your focus with cue words—single words or phrases that act like keyboard shortcuts to direct attention in a more positive or facilitative way. Repeat motivational cue words to trigger the emotions you would prefer to be experiencing (for instance, "calm" or "confident"). Instructional cue words direct your focus to your body and your form, improving your physical execution ("knees soft" or "chest up").

Note that there are also cue words that can unintentionally feed the monster. This can happen when you label your injured body parts. If you find yourself referring to your "good knee" (or ankle, or shoulder) versus your "bad knee," consider the message you're feeding your brain. Every morsel you can throw to the athlete instead of the monster adds up over time.

IMAGERY

Imagery—also referred to as visualization or mental rehearsal—involves the ability to create and recreate images in your mind. For many people, this takes a significant amount of practice. However, once you develop this skill, it will remain a powerful mental training tool to have in your arsenal. We talked about this a bit in Chapter 3 with the idea of mental contrasting, and in the Healing Visions drill on page 73, but it's worth exploring explicitly as a source of fuel for your athlete.

With recent advances in neuroimaging, we now know that many of the same neural pathways are used in both imagery and actual visual perception. The only difference is that with imagery, your motor neurons don't engage, so you're not actually going through the motions. Still, you've carried out powerful neural groundwork for how you'll react and respond later on when you are performing the actions. From imagining your body healing to seeing yourself back in competitive action, imagery can be an important part of your mental training throughout your recovery. You'll feel more motivated if you see where you are headed, and more confident when you're cleared to return. After all, you've been practicing in your mind, even if your body isn't quite there yet. As well as the Seeing Is Believing drill on pages 157–158, you can try using Healing Visions on page 73 and Mental Movies on pages 180–181.

USE CURIOSITY AS A CATALYST

If you start to pay attention to the body language, thoughts, and imagery you use each day, you'll notice plenty of opportunities to feed your athlete instead of your monster. Sometimes, you need a bit of a push over the hump from self-defeating patterns to productive thoughts and behaviors. Don't let this upset or frustrate you—it's challenging to change those habits.

One way to shift your mindset is to cultivate curiosity about your injury. When you can tap into an authentic yearning to explore and understand, you'll start to feel an emotional shift from being a victim of your injury to wanting to learn about it. Instead of recoiling in fear or anger, you lean in, hoping to engage in and derive the most benefit from each step of the process. Essentially, you can transform yourself into a student of your injury—and, indeed, of the entire injury experience.

Curiosity creates a sense of separation, so you can witness your injury objectively rather than being consumed by it. You shift from "Why is this happening to me?" to "What exactly is happening here?" Though it seems counterintuitive at first, this detachment actually makes it easier to take positive steps toward recovery.

We hope this entire book stokes your curiosity for how you can get through your injury, and even for what you can take away from it. If you're having trouble getting there, see if you can nudge yourself by setting up a mini-experiment. Pick a mental drill in this book that intrigues you—even a little bit—or if all else fails, just open to a random page and flip to the first drill you find. Do it once or twice, and see if it makes a difference in how you feel. Not all the exercises will work for everyone at every point in the process, but by testing one out and noticing your response, you automatically shift from a critical mode to one of curiosity.

Let's take some more looks at how feeding your athlete works in real life.

Winning the inner game

Carrie Tollefson, the Olympic runner we met in Chapter 2, spent her fair share of time rehabbing from injuries, including coming back from surgery to remove a benign tumor from her foot and recovering from stress fractures and muscle tears. She had her dark moments—times when she doubted whether she could continue—but never wallowed in them for long. "I didn't let myself go too negative because it just wasn't in me to go there," she said.

Visualization helped her feed her athlete during challenging times. So, too, did positive self-talk. She'd stare at herself in the mirror while pedaling on the elliptical and think: "You are one of the best in the world" and "No one's working harder than you."

- - -

Pitcher Tanner Biwer was a middle-schooler playing basketball when he first slipped and hurt his hip—an injury that lingered throughout his high-school and college baseball career at Marian University in Fond du Lac, Wisconsin. Finally, he wound up having surgery in college. Doctors told him he had a congenital hip defect that, over the years, had caused him to tear his labrum and wear away nearly all his cartilage. Recovery from the surgery was even more difficult than he'd expected—instead of three weeks of being non-weight-bearing, as he'd been told beforehand, his surgeon determined he'd need six weeks on crutches and then another month and a half of rehab.

His athletic trainer, who happened to be a physical therapist, kept him motivated by developing a solid plan for his return. Biwer used visualization both during rehab and when he returned to the field, even mining his nighttime visions for glimpses of his successful rebound. "I would have dreams where I was running and I was full-blown bouncy, pitching well and everything," he said. "I really took that unconscious entity and brought it into my day-to-day work."

He combined that with powerful body positioning and physical preparation, especially before a game. While his teammates might have used music and trash talk, Biwer knew what it would take for him to get into his groove. "I would take a lot of time to do an extensive dynamic warm-up and stretch and visualize while I'm doing those things," he said. "I'd think, 'What do I want my pitches to look like?' It was important for me to sit back and be with me before I got into the physical aspects of my performance."

And then there were the cue words—these helped him recover both from physical injury and from intermittent cases of the yips, where he'd find himself mentally unable to perform well. He always wrote a key phrase on his cap. "I'd take my hat off and I'd just read the words: 'Breathe and focus.' It brought me back to my task at hand and what I needed to do."

\- - -

British runner Perri Shakes-Drayton's injury experience played out on an international stage. In the 2013 World Championships in Moscow, during the finals of the 400-meter hurdles, the Olympian tore a knee ligament and damaged the cartilage surrounding it, requiring surgery. The days afterward were dark, she said in an interview. She'd always seen injury as a sign of weakness, and now that it had struck her, she felt lost and confused.

Although she'd always continue to run, she knew immediately she'd move away from hurdles. But as she prepared to return to running, at first she couldn't bear to be anywhere near her sport. As she began to recover, she'd watch others' performances and start to gain confidence. "I was like, I've run faster than that," she said. "I look back at videos now, and I'm like, wow, I was awesome. I *am* awesome." She took inspiration from other athletes who've made incredible comebacks, including gymnast Asha Philip and hurdler Lolo Jones. She would read encouraging books—one of her favorites was called, fittingly enough, *You Are Awesome*—and she turned to shopping and music for emotional lifts.

And she surrounded herself with people who believed in her. "Mentally, you have to be so tough, because people will say things and kind of doubt you. You don't need that—you need people to focus you. My coach [Chris Zah] is a key player in that; he was at the hospital appointments, my rehab appointments. He was there, he would travel. Every time I made a bit of progress, he would make me feel stronger, and that is what you need."

After a stint on the popular TV show *Dancing on Ice*, Shakes-Drayton returned to competition, and was part of Great Britain's silver medal–winning 4x400-meter relay team at the 2017 World Championships. "I was buzzing—like, wow, I'm back," she said. "I'm more appreciative of it because you never know what's around the corner."

THE 80/20 RULE

In the 1890s, the curiosity of Italian economist Vilfredo Pareto led him to observe that 80% of the land in Italy was owned by 20% of the population. Since then, the Pareto Principle, or the 80/20 rule, has been applied to many different areas, including business and economics, computers and software, even clothing. The premise revolves around an inherent imbalance between input and output—the fact that 20% of the effort leads to 80% of the reward, that 20% of the tasks produce 80% of the achievement (or, in the case of clothing, that we tend to wear a select 20% of our wardrobe 80% of the time).

If we suppose that this principle applies to your mindset and your rehab and recovery, here are some key questions to ask yourself:

◆ Which 20% of my daily life is causing me 80% of my daily stress?
◆ Which 20% of my time spent leads to 80% of my joy?
◆ Which 20% of my friends provide me with 80% of my happiness?
◆ Which 20% of my monster thoughts are creating 80% of my mental anguish?

Taking the time to understand these answers can essentially offer you a nutrition plan to feed your athlete. Really sit down with it—your answers might surprise you. By figuring out what fuels your stress and anguish and your happiness and joy, you can then consciously choose to focus your energy on what ignites you instead of what drains you. You can work smarter, not harder, aligning your time, efforts, and mental energy with the emotions that will allow you to reach your long-term goals.

YOUR QUICK FOUR-STEP CONFIDENCE BOOST

When you feed your athlete instead of your monster, you also build confidence— another key mental skill that allows you to rebound. We often talk about confidence as something you have inside you, but in fact it's also a skill you can practice and improve.

While overall confidence serves you well in the recovery process, what's even more important is a specific type of confidence called self-efficacy—scientific lingo for your belief in your own ability to succeed in a given situation. Athletes with higher levels of self-efficacy are more likely to follow their rehabilitation program (and remember from Chapter 3 that athletes who follow their rehabilitation program are more likely to have successful outcomes and a successful recovery).

If you feed your athlete regularly with positive body language, thoughts, and imagery, your confidence is more likely to stay healthy too. Still, you might face moments where your self-efficacy wavers—where you're questioning if you have what it takes to get through the task or the day ahead of you, let alone your entire rehab and recovery.

When this happens, first stop and take a breath. Then, go through the following four steps. Think of them as a quick infusion of high-dose vitamins— a nutritious supplement for your psyche.

1. *Normalize the event.* Injury isolates—at times, you may feel like you're the only person on the planet going through this. Remind yourself that injury is a natural if undesirable part of the athletic journey, and that it provokes a roller coaster of often negative emotions. Resist the urge to judge yourself for what is happening or to over-personalize the experience. Drills to use: Emotion Decoder (see pages 28–29); Go FAR (see page 46); Compare with Compassion (see pages 158–159).
2. *Reappraise and reframe.* Think about taking a photo for Instagram, and then applying a filter and a frame. These steps can change the

picture entirely. In the same way, can you look at your challenge differently, in a way that moves you forward rather than trapping you in anger, disappointment, and a feeling of being overwhelmed? Drills to use: Yes, And… (see pages 75–76); Found in Translation (see pages 135–136); Funhouse Mirror (see pages 48–49).

3. *Cultivate hope.* The rehab and recovery process can test the mental endurance of even the most determined athlete. But even when you feel you've reached the end of your rope, you can choose determination instead of despair. This is when you need to start feeding your athlete with positive self-talk, such as "I will get through this" or "I still believe. I still have faith." You might also reach out for emotional support at this time. Drills to try: Build Your Team (see page 133); Injury Mantras (see pages 70–71); Athlete Affirmations (see page 180).

4. *Seek lessons and opportunities.* Here's where that curiosity comes in again. Now that you know what's happening is normal, are able to view it from a couple of different angles, and have hope that you can get through it—what can you learn? How can you ultimately be better for having gone through this experience? Drills to try: Obstacles to Opportunities (see pages 46–47); Redefine Success (see page 70); Hero's Journey (see pages 74–75).

Aiming for the rebound is a choice that you alone can make. No one else gets to choose how your injury defines you—only *you*.

The Chinese philosopher Chuang Tzu said, "The road is made by people walking on it; things are so because they are called so. What makes them so? Making them so makes them so. What makes them not so? Making them not so makes them not so."

In other words, whatever you decide is true is true. When you feed your athlete, you are creating a road of resilience and perseverance through your injury experience. You get to create the meaning of this journey. The road is called so because you have called it so.

Rebuilding an athlete

British triathlete Alistair Robinson was on a training ride on April 21, 2014, on a route not far from his home in Keswick, Cumbria, when he crashed into a vehicle. He has no recollection of what happened—his memory stops about a mile before the accident site. His injuries included a fractured skull, nine broken vertebrae, and a severe concussion, and required a seven-hour operation, permanent plates in his back, and three months in a halo brace to support his neck.

Afterward, Robinson thought long and hard about whether he wanted to return to the sport. Through introspection and many long, deep conversations with his partner, Robinson determined he did, not because of external pressures but because he was still curious about his untapped potential. "The accident was even more intriguing because that's almost the equivalent of writing off a car—no one would try to repair that car," he told us in an interview. "Nothing but the human body, when put through that, could come back and maybe even come back better."

He first lined up again at Ironman 70.3 Barcelona in May 2015, just a year and a week after the crash. He finished 25th in 4 hours and 40 minutes. He did a few more races and even began surpassing his previous times on the swim and run, and won the Ben Nevis Braveheart Tri that October. But soon, the lingering effects of his injuries began to interfere with his training in ways that he felt limited his performances. So, he pulled back from racing and redirected his time and energy into addressing these issues like ongoing spasms in his neck (and also to pursue coaching, with a focus on assisting older athletes and those who've gone through traumatic injuries). The lost mobility in his upper back meant he needed to work more on chest flexibility to avoid pinched, hunched shoulders after the bike and swim. The edges of the metal fusing his vertebrae stab and scar his muscles when he trains for too long, a problem he's still figuring out how to solve. He stays motivated by curiosity, by the intellectual and physical challenges of putting the broken pieces of an athlete back together again.

To make sure he feeds his athlete and not his monster, Robinson has made a few adjustments. He has unfollowed on social media some of the athletes he used to compete against, so that he's not tempted to begrudge them any of their current successes. (Use the Compare with Compassion drill on pages 158–159 to assess your own interactions, both online and in-person.) He realizes it's not worthwhile to try to figure out what happened during the accident, so when he catches his mind wandering in that direction, he gently redirects it (the Thoughtstopper drill on pages 156–157 is another way to regain control).

In a way, the whole experience has offered Robinson a release, a liberation. He came to triathlon relatively late and always felt he was years behind his rivals. "After the injury, I don't feel any time pressure anymore. I feel like if everything goes to plan and I still want it, I can be faster at 39, 40, as an Ironman athlete than I've ever been in my life," he said. "Personally, I think I've got way more potential as an athlete and a person now than I had before it happened."

Did you catch the rebound? Robinson bounced when he channeled his curiosity about how well he could perform after his injury. He bounced again when he chose to feed his athlete a steady diet of positive thoughts and social media posts.

JUST THE FACTS

- Thoughts have tremendous power to steer your recovery in a positive direction—or to derail it completely.
- Your own self-talk—the inner dialogue and constant chatter running through your head—plays just as big a role as the words of others, if not a bigger one.
- Your inner athlete and your inner monster are vying for your attention, and you are the one who decides which of them will get it.
- Thoughts and emotions can cause excess stress and have an influence over your behavior. You have the power to influence those attitudes and mindsets.
- Your inner athlete can thrive on a relatively varied diet; you can feed it with body language, thoughts, and imagery.
- When you can cultivate curiosity about your injury, you'll feel an emotional shift from being a victim of your injury to wanting to learn about it.
- Confidence isn't just something you have inside you—it's a skill you can practice and improve.
- When you feed your athlete, you are creating a road of resilience and perseverance through your injury experience.

MENTAL SKILLS AND DRILLS

How can you use your mind to heal your muscles like Bernd Zangerl, find motivating cue words and rituals like Tanner Biwer, seek external driving forces like Perri Shakes-Drayton, even view your entire injury process as an intellectual opportunity like Alistair Robinson? The following drills provide critical guidance and practice in fostering the confidence and resilience you need to rebound.

MENTAL DRILL: CHART YOUR CONFIDENCE

Understand and influence the factors that affect your confidence level.

Mental Skills
Level 1, Rookie: Confidence, Focus, Motivation
Level 2, All-Star: Self-Awareness
Level 3, Hall of Fame: Resilience

This drill boosts your self-efficacy, that super-specific type of confidence we discussed as being critical to the rebound process. Think about a task you have ahead of you and ask yourself, "How confident do I feel in my ability to do this right now?" On a scale of one to ten, one being zero confidence and ten being zero doubt, how would you rank your level of confidence in this moment? (you'll find a template to map this out in the workbook from www.injuredathletesclub.com.)

Once you assign your confidence a number (and no half-points here, don't overthink it; simply commit to a full number), ask yourself: "Why didn't I rank myself one point lower?" Then ask: "What would need to be different in order to rank myself one point higher?" Answering these questions will reinforce the confidence you already have, as well as pinpoint actions you can take to increase your feelings of confidence and move yourself one point forward. Don't worry about getting to a ten, just focus on what you need to do to take it one step further. Anytime you feel anxious, unsure, doubtful, do this mental drill, and chart your confidence.

MENTAL DRILL: FLIP THE SCRIPT

Craft versions of your injury story that build rather than deplete your confidence and strength.

Mental Skills
Level 1, Rookie: Confidence, Focus, Stress Management
Level 2, All-Star: Attitude, Communication, Emotional Intelligence

One of the unique stressors of being injured is having to face telling your injury story over and over and over again. Often, this evokes dread and turns into a trigger that ignites emotions like annoyance, anger, shame, guilt, and sadness. However, you can flip the script and craft your injury story in a way that's empowering instead of draining.

In fact, you might even have two scripts—one that includes the full injury story you tell the people you're closest to, and one abridged version that you can tell everyone else. When someone asks what happened, you have the power to choose which script to share.

Actually write out your scripts, practice saying them, and notice how you feel when you do. One important question to ask yourself is: "How do *I* want to feel about my injury right now?" When people ask about your injury, you might feel like you're supposed to take on the emotion they're projecting onto you. But you have the power—and the responsibility—to tell the story in a way that evokes your desired feelings.

So instead of:

"I don't know what happened. It was just a freak accident. I'm so upset. I have no idea when or if I'll ever be able to play again. Can we talk about something else?"

Try:

"I was having a great game and I really went after it. When I came down I just landed wrong. It sucks and it's definitely something I wish I wasn't dealing with, but I'm focused on my new goals and getting stronger every day. How are things going for you?"

Remember: You are the author and *you choose* how to tell your story.

MENTAL DRILL: THOUGHTSTOPPER

Visualize blocking and replacing each negative thought.

Mental Skills
Level 1, Rookie: Focus, Stress Management
Level 2, All-Star: Emotional Intelligence, Visualization

You can't simply shut out negative emotions without honoring them—but there are times when thoughts and feelings that aren't serving you linger long after you've paid them their due. Negative emotions can become repetitive or automatic; that's when they truly start feeding your monster instead of your athlete. If you've tried labeling your negative emotions and even speaking them out loud and they haven't gone away—or they come back—you might have to take things a step further and use visualization to block them.

Imagine you found a dark and dusty glass bottle with a cork on top. When you pull the cork out, an ear-piercing sound escapes from the bottle. So you quickly shove the cork back in, stopping the noise immediately. For this mental drill, you're going to come up with your own visual thoughtstopper. As well as putting a cork back in a bottle, consider:

◆ Seeing a bright red stop sign or stoplight
◆ Having a bucket of ice water dumped over your head
◆ Pulling the emergency brake on a freight train.

Whatever you come up with, choose a powerful visual for stopping your unwanted automatic thought in its tracks. Employ it when you need it—then take the opportunity to replace that thought with one that feeds your athlete. Over time, you'll find it easier and easier to choke the negative neural pathway and redirect yourself toward recovery.

MENTAL DRILL: SEEING IS BELIEVING

Use imagery to help "feed your athlete."

Mental Skills
Level 1, Rookie: Confidence, Focus, Motivation, Stress Management
Level 2, All-Star: Visualization

Imagery exercises visually feed your athlete by allowing you to see in your mind what you want to come true in your life. Depending on where you are in the rehab and recovery process, you might choose to focus on a different element. There are four main categories of imagery:

◆ *Healing:* Picture your body recovering. This could be a literal physiological image—bones strengthening, torn ligaments repairing—or a symbolic depiction, such as light or warmth in the injured area.
◆ *Relaxing:* Calming visualizations balance out your stress response—maybe it's an image of your favorite restful vacation, a place or situation in which you feel entirely safe and secure, or a progressive relaxation, where you imagine letting go of tension in your body from your toes to your head (or vice versa). This can also be used to reduce pain.
◆ *Motivational:* Give yourself an energizing boost during times when you're struggling with a long recovery or with a lack of desire to go to

rehab or to train. Picture yourself being mentally tough, confident, or focused during a difficult situation.

◆ *Performance:* Picture yourself successfully performing a specific task—say, a rehab exercise—or imagine yourself in competition.

Once you choose an area of focus, write a script that you will then record and listen to on a regular basis. To make the most of your imagery exercises, focus on:

◆ *Vividness:* To create high-definition images in your mind, make your script as descriptive as you can. Add in elements from all five senses (taste, touch, smell, sight, and sound). Adding the emotions you want to be feeling increases vividness as well.

◆ *Controllability:* Start as simply as you need to in order to control the images you're creating. Visualization is a skill that improves over time. If your thoughts start to go rogue, pull back. You're using the same preparatory neural pathways as if you were actually living out the experience; maintaining control keeps you on the pathway that feeds your athlete.

◆ *Recording:* Eventually, you might be able to visualize without the script or the recording, but it's incredibly helpful to have them at first. When recording the script, be sure to read slowly and pause longer than feels natural between sentences. If you feel uncomfortable hearing your own voice on the recording, try having a friend, teammate, or family member record it for you instead (or even use your computer voice).

If you don't want to create your own script—or if you want some inspiration to start—check out the Headspace app, under the "sport" section. The Recovery and Rehab packs are among our favorites!

MENTAL DRILL: COMPARE WITH COMPASSION

Explore when comparison helps and when it holds you back.

Mental Skills
Level 1, Rookie: Confidence, Stress Management
Level 2, All-Star: Attitude
Level 3, Hall of Fame: Discipline, Generosity

When you compare your injury journey and recovery timeline with another athlete's, you walk a fine line between feeding your monster and feeding your athlete. On one hand, commiserating with someone going through injury—especially the same injury as yours—can give you motivation and hope or provide you with information about what to expect and what is possible. Hearing about other injured athletes who have recovered from their injuries and successfully returned to competition, or about athletes who were able to remain positive and resilient in the face of needing to choose a different activity after recovering from injury, can be a potent way to start feeling confident in your own ability to do the same thing (that's one reason we're writing this book for you, and including lots of athletes' stories).

However, if you start comparing their journey with your journey and internalizing it in a negative way, you've tipped over to feeding your monster. Keep a log of comparisons, including how they make you feel, and whether they feed your monster or your athlete. When you do find a situation that feeds your monster, ask yourself how you could avoid it or see it through a different lens next time (You can find a blank chart to make these notes in the workbook at www.injuredathletesclub.com.)

I COMPARED MYSELF WITH...	I FELT...	DID I FEED MY MONSTER OR MY ATHLETE?
An athlete who recovered from the same injury very quickly.	Inspired by the thought that I could do the same.	Athlete
An athlete who recovered from the same injury very quickly.	Discouraged that I wasn't moving along at the same rate.	Monster
An athlete who took a long time to recover from a different injury.	Overwhelmed with despair.	Monster
An athlete who took a long time to recover from a different injury.	Empathy for what that athlete's gone through and gratitude that I'm on a different path.	Athlete
My teammates who don't have injuries.	Angry and jealous that I have to sit out.	Monster
My teammates who don't have injuries.	Motivated to rejoin them—and to help them in another way while I'm sidelined.	Athlete

MENTAL DRILL: PEN PALS

Write a letter to your injured body part—and a response.

Mental Skills
Level 1, Rookie: Stress Management
Level 2, All-Star: Communication
Level 3, Hall of Fame: Psychological Flexibility

Yes, you read that right—you're going to personify your injury, turning it into an independent being who can put pen to paper. You might think this sounds strange, but we'd strongly encourage you to give it a try. Creating a separate persona for your injury depersonalizes what is happening to you, offering you a different lens through which to view and understand your rehab and recovery process.

Step one is to give your injury a name—one different from "my bad knee" or "my bad shoulder," terms that subconsciously feed your monster. (One of Carrie's injured athletes, Sonoma State University tennis player Jordyn Kearney, named her knee "Ryan.") Don't rush this part; sit with the idea and something will likely come to you. You may be surprised to find that the name you come up with will actually become a term of endearment for your injury.

In this exercise you will be writing two letters. Make sure you carve out some uninterrupted time to dedicate to this mental drill. Sometimes it helps to change locations, especially if you're struggling to get started. Take a hike or go to a park with a notebook and try writing while you're in a different environment. Or you can head to your home court or field, wherever you usually practice, preferably during a time when you can be there alone.

The first letter is from you to your injury, expressing any thoughts and feelings you'd want to share. Don't censor yourself. Be OK with whatever comes out. Don't analyze as you write—just write. If you're stuck on how to start, here are some questions to consider:

- How are you feeling about your injury right now?
- How do you view the situation overall?
- What unanswered questions remain?
- What fears do you have?
- What do you need to hear from your injury?

For the second letter, embody that personification of your injury. How does Martha (or Skippy, or Ryan, or whatever name you choose) respond to your letter? Again, here are some prompts if you need them:

- How does your injury view the situation?
- What is the reason for your injury?
- Why is this an important part of your greater athletic journey?
- What emotions does your injury feel for you?
- What advice does your injury have for you?

Even just writing the first letter can be very powerful, but we encourage you to try the second letter as well. Notice how you feel afterward. You may find the response to be quite extraordinary.

CHAPTER 8

NOW WHAT?

"My body is stronger. My mind is stronger. And I notice I have so much joy when I try to do everything to 100 percent. This injury made me realize how much I enjoy soccer and how big it is in my life."
—*Chicago Fire forward Michael de Leeuw*

Being cleared to compete again is a huge milestone, but it doesn't mean the recovery process is over. Ongoing patience and diligence will aid your re-entry and help you anticipate and cope with the range of obstacles and fears arising during this period. Mental skills build your confidence as you get ready to return to your sport. And if you're altering your athletic endeavors—either because of your physical limitations or because you've made a conscious choice to step away from your sport—you can use them to cope with the transition and direct your future path.

The path back to the pitch

For ten long months in 2017 and 2018, soccer fans in Chicago had missed the Lion's roar. Chicago Fire forward Michael de Leeuw—whose last name is Dutch for lion, hence the nickname—had been out since

September 2017. A collision in the twenty-sixth minute of a game against the New York Red Bulls ruptured his left ACL.

Upon realizing he'd be out for at least the rest of the season, de Leeuw struggled at first, he explained during an interview with us. He feared for his future and his livelihood—he was already thirty, with a new baby, and a contract up in a year. But he didn't allow his anxieties to consume him. After three or four days to adjust to his new reality, de Leeuw channeled a Dutch idiom: "je hoofd boven water houden," which roughly translates to always rising up above the water instead of sinking.

He had surgery in November 2017, then stayed in Chicago over the holidays, logging lonely hours daily at the club doing his rehab exercises—stepping off boxes, walking slowly on the treadmill, and pushing and pulling against elastic bands.

Soon, though, he had company. His rookie teammate, midfielder Djordje Mihailovic, tore his ACL a month later, and the two recovered together. "I took Djordje a little bit under my wing," de Leeuw said. What Mihailovic might not have realized, though, was how much he helped his mentor, too. Each time de Leeuw imparted wisdom and motivation to the younger player—telling him, for example, to push hard but to be realistic about his timeline—the lessons sank in more deeply for the elder player, too.

Each milestone propelled de Leeuw forward—the first time he bent his knee, the day he could finally walk and sleep without a brace (choose your own milestones to celebrate with the Redefine Success drill on page 70). As winter became spring and summer, he began running outdoors, then practicing on the field.

The last two months actually felt the most difficult of all. Most times, he felt hungry, eager to return to the game he loved—in June 2018, for example, after he came back to practice with the team, trainers had to hold him back from completing every drill and exercise. Other days, however, doubt flashed through his mind—would his repaired joint truly withstand the demands he'd have to place on it? (Use the Chart Your Confidence drill on page 155 to identify—and address—your apprehensions.)

In the same way that he'd worked hard in rehab, de Leeuw devised a plan to counter these fears. He placed his trust in his trainer and medical team, knowing they shared the same goals as he did, as well as the expertise to help him reach them. By slowly building up to full team practices, including a training tournament in July, he developed faith that his knee would hold up when he ran, kicked, cut, or stopped (more on using this step-by-step approach in the Anxiety Pyramid drill on pages 113–114). And to reduce his risk of hurting anything else, he focused diligently on recovery, adding swimming to his routine and spending every spare minute at home in contrast baths or recovery boots.

Finally, on August 12, 2018, the day de Leeuw had worked so hard for arrived. The Red Bulls returned to the Fire's home field, Toyota Park. De Leeuw came in as a second-half substitution, spent seventeen minutes playing and even got a few touches on the ball. The time passed quickly. He knew there was more work to do—further fitness training and skills to continue fine-tuning after a year off—but he felt grateful for the opportunity to move forward. At the end of the year, he signed a new contract with FC Emmen, back home in the Netherlands.

Did you catch the rebound? De Leeuw bounced when he allowed himself a period of sadness, then moved on mentally to begin rehab. He bounced again when he chose to focus on what he could do to boost his confidence as he returned to competition rather than succumb to his doubts and fears of re-injury.

CLIMBING THE LAST BIG MOUNTAIN

Way back in Chapter 1, we discussed the roller coaster of emotions you're likely to experience post-injury. When you first get hurt, all you can think about is how frustrated you are at being sidelined and how desperately you want to return. You've undoubtedly faced some challenging moments since then, but on the whole, you may have noticed your emotions generally becoming more positive as your physical status improves.

This balance between feeling better physically and feeling better mentally often shifts again as you prepare to return to activity. Research—as well as experience—tells us the closer you get to medical clearance, the more anxious you may become. Even if you've been diligent about feeding your athlete with confidence-building thoughts and actions, as we describe in Chapter 7, you might find yourself unwittingly feeding your monster of negativity with renewed worries and doubts. The dreaded "what-ifs" you'd once banished start to re-enter your mind as you focus on all of the unknowns.

Even when your doctors, therapists, and trainers give you official medical clearance, you can still feel the fear, thinking, "Am I really ready?" Often, athletes find their bodies are physically primed before their minds are fully prepared to return to action. The good news, which you'll know if you've worked your way through this book, is that diligent attention to your mental rehabilitation in addition to your physical rehabilitation makes it far more likely that your mind and body will sync up at this stage. Even if you're just starting to focus on mental training, there is a lot you can do at this point to address the specific psychological challenges of returning to higher levels of training intensity and, eventually, to competition.

At this stage of the game, four main concerns often surface:

◆ Can I return to my pre-injury ability?
◆ Will people perceive me as weak or unfit?
◆ Do I still have a place on this team?
◆ Will I overcome my fear of re-injury?

For many of you, the fear of re-injury is the concern dominating your mind at this point—it's the item listed at the very top of your Anxiety Pyramid from Chapter 5. That's such a huge deal, so we'll delve into it more deeply later in the chapter (and if you want to go straight there, flip to pages 113–114). For now, let's look at the other three issues, their underlying causes, and some potential solutions—including drills from earlier in the book that you might want to revisit and update for this new stage.

CAN I RETURN TO MY PRE-INJURY ABILITY?

As you start to ramp up your training intensity and test out your injured body part, it's natural to wonder whether you'll be the same athlete you were before your injury. Your questions might include:

◆ Is my body going to be able to handle the same workload?
◆ Will I be able to cut and run the way I did before?
◆ Am I going to fatigue more quickly and not have the endurance I need?
◆ Will I still be able to achieve the goals I set out for myself before I got injured?

These concerns arise because you haven't been able to fully test your skills. The possibility of coming back and not being able to play to the same level you were performing at pre-injury is yet another threat to your athletic identity—which, as we've discussed, usually takes a big blow throughout the rehab process. Dwelling too much on this question may lead you to prolong your recovery to avoid sub-optimal performances, or even to unwisely accelerate your timeline in a desperate hunt for answers.

THE CURE

Keep reminding yourself that fitness and technical skills will return with time. Aim to gauge your feelings of success not in terms of what you were capable of doing before your injury, but instead on the basis of where your body is right now. Be patient and set goals specific to your current fitness level—celebrate when you achieve them, then continue to reach to the next step. Notice if you feel different when you shift your focus from what you've lost to what you've gained through this experience. Consider coming up with a new set of mantras. Try: *I'm ready. I've done the work. I'm a stronger, smarter athlete.*

Mental Drills to Revisit & Revise

MENTAL DRILL	CHAPTER	PAGE NO.
Grab Your Goals	3	72–73
Injury Mantras	3	70–71
Feel and Focus	4	89
R&R	5	111–112
Chart Your Confidence	7	155
Pen Pals	7	160–161

WILL PEOPLE PERCEIVE ME AS WEAK OR UNFIT?

As an athlete, you spend a good portion of your competitive career reading the reactions of your teammates and opponents. Depending on your level and your sport, you may have fans and financial supporters as well. As you return, you may become so focused on what other people are thinking about your performance that it becomes a major distraction. These thoughts are common: *Will my coach and my teammates trust me to get the job done? Will my sponsors drop me?* You don't want to let down the people who are counting on you and who believe in your ability to come back—nor do you want to show weakness to your opponents or detractors.

THE CURE

There are two sides to this story: others' perceptions and your own reactions. You have far more control over the second than the first, so let's start there. Keep reminding yourself of what you've already achieved. Step back and look at your progress on a continuum—you are much closer to the end of your journey than the beginning. Consider the hours you've put into both physically and mentally recovering; even as your fitness and technique return, you're now also armed with mental toughness and specific skills, such as visualization, to enhance your future performances.

Shifting to this mindset will imbue you with confidence that transmits to those around you—after all, part of what they'll assess is your attitude. If you're negative or pessimistic about your status and progress, they're far more likely to pick that up and believe it. Another step you might consider is giving your coaches and sponsors progress reports on your recovery, with specific focus on the milestones you've surpassed and the realistic goals you've set for the days and weeks to come.

Mental Drills to Revisit & Revise

MENTAL DRILL	CHAPTER	PAGE NO.
Emotion Decoder	1	28–29
Sidelined SWOT	1	30–31
Go FAR	2	46
Stop/Start/Continue	3	71
In/Out of Control	4	88
Found in Translation	6	135

DO I STILL HAVE A PLACE ON THIS TEAM?

Injury can leave you with the impression that your peers are moving ahead with their fitness and ability, leaving you in the dust (and possibly even forgetting who you are altogether). If you're on a team, you might start to wonder if you're going to get cut or if the person who stepped into your position will continue once you return. Off the field or court, you can also perceive a breakdown in your social connection to the team; your teammates continued bonding while you were isolated, out of the loop.

THE CURE

Remind yourself that you've been a member of the team all along, even if you had to train and practice in a different location for a while. Recall from Chapter 2 that you can hold two seemingly opposing views at the same time: It's OK to simultaneously feel excited for your teammate who is starting in your place and disappointed for your own loss, or elated that your team is doing well while also angry and upset that you've missed part of the experience. Consider how to judge a successful first practice or competition back—the measures may be very different from what they were before your injury. Know that your contribution to your team right now consists of making your recovery your sport and coming back mentally and physically strong.

Mental Drills to Revisit & Revise

MENTAL DRILL	CHAPTER	PAGE NO.
Obstacles to Opportunities	2	46–47
Bad News/Good News	2	47–48
Redefine Success	3	70
Time-Travel Log	4	87–88
Build Your Team	6	133
Compare with Compassion	7	158–159

HURRY UP AND WAIT

Since each athlete's injury journey is different, you might not be dealing with these precise concerns, but if any of them resonate with you, it's important to address them rather than sweep them under the rug. If you don't, they may lead you to return to your sport before you're truly ready, mentally and physically.

Other reasons you might return prematurely include:

◆ Your own excitement, if you're feeling strong and ready. Often, when athletes think of mental toughness, they conjure an image of working hard or pushing through pain. But when you're returning to training and competition after an injury, sometimes mental toughness means holding back rather than gutting through.

◆ External pressures. You might rush because you're relying on income from your sport, you have an important tryout or competition, or you fear you'll lose sponsorships. Maybe your coach and your teammates ask how you are with a subtle (or not-so-subtle) underlying context of, "When are you coming back? We really need you!" Even your family and friends might inadvertently add pressure, knowing how tough it's been for you to spend time away from your sport. Note that these pressures may be real, but it's also possible that your views on them are skewed as you filter others' statements and actions through a lens biased by fear or eagerness.

There's always some guesswork involved in planning a successful return to training and competition, but athletes tend to do best when they work together with their medical team to devise a thought-out plan. Every athlete who has returned too soon and suffered additional setbacks will tell you it's not worth it. In this case, sprinting to the finish might move the finish line farther out of reach. Getting both your body and your mind on the same page sets you up for a successful comeback.

Of course, if you do move ahead and find you've pushed too soon or too far, avoid the trap of fearing you're heading back to square one. Just as they are at every other point during your rebound, setbacks are a normal part of the process of defining and redefining your limits. Recovery isn't completely linear, and you'll face ups and downs all along the way. When you encounter setbacks—no matter what the cause—at this stage, remember how you've handled them all along the way. View them not as signs of failure, but as opportunities to bounce even higher.

BUT—DON'T DRAG THINGS OUT

While some athletes fight the temptation to rush back before they're ready, others experience the opposite, prolonging their athletic return. This is more likely to occur if:

◆ You were feeling pressure and/or burnout before your injury
◆ You are enjoying secondary gains
◆ You are afraid of getting re-injured.

FEELING PRESSURE AND/OR BURNOUT
BEFORE YOUR INJURY

If you were experiencing anxiety and pressure before getting injured, you may actually have found yourself feeling some relief at getting a break from your sport. Or if you were feeling burnout before your injury, you may be at a crossroads where your injury has allowed you to ask yourself the question: "Do I really want to go back?" We'll address this question in depth at the end of the chapter.

ENJOYING SECONDARY GAINS

Secondary gains are positive consequences of injury, such as increased attention and support from significant others. Some may feel a sense of relief at being removed from the stress of intense training schedules and the pressures of performance. Consciously or subconsciously, you might fear these perks will disappear when you're healthy.

FEAR OF RE-INJURY

After your body's failed you once, it's only normal to experience ongoing worries about your fragility. Your brain has realized—perhaps for the first time—that your body is vulnerable. In addition, you're ramping up your intensity, testing out your injured body part and your overall fitness in ways you haven't since you got hurt. You're now on high alert, watching out for warning signs that you'll become injured again.

While some caution is warranted, your brain often tends to overcompensate, dialing up your vigilance to the point where it's detrimental rather than beneficial. The amount of excess fear you feel can depend on some of the same situational and personal factors that were involved in your initial response to your injury, such as whether you've been hurt before and the amount of support you've had in your comeback. More severe injuries often result in greater fears when you return, in part because of how long you've been away from your sport, and also because you may be getting closer to doing the thing that caused your injury in the first place. These feelings can intensify in the lead-up to your return, but often linger even after you've been back for a while.

It's a cruel twist, but these fears of re-injury themselves actually increase your risk of getting hurt again, whether it's via a similar mechanism or to a different part of your body. Why? Back in Chapter 5, we discussed the stress response.

When you encounter a situation that potentially threatens your well-being, your brain kicks off a physiological response with real physical effects, some of which can contribute to re-injury. For example:

- Your muscles tense up
- Your coordination decreases
- You lose your balance
- Your peripheral vision fades
- You fatigue more quickly
- You can't concentrate.

Anxiety about re-injury can just plain take your head out of the game. If you're preoccupied with fears and doubts, your focus stays there instead of tuning into your surrounding environment. You might miss important cues to prevent a collision, a breakdown of form, or some other situation in which injury may occur.

Of course, this assumes that you actually make it back to training and competition in the first place. If you haven't taken the time to build up your confidence as you've built up your strength, you may choose to keep yourself out of practice or competition, even if your body is ready and you've received medical clearance. If fear is holding you back from competing and you are feeling frustrated, as though your mind is the only thing standing in your way—know that you can work through this. You may just need some time to build your mental fitness back up to the level of your physical fitness.

First, acknowledge your fears—but don't dwell on them. Know you are experiencing a normal emotional and physiological reaction. Your brain is taking steps to protect your body. Fearing re-injury isn't a sign of weakness or that you're not mentally tough—so just "sucking it up" won't work. Even if you haven't had this fear with previous injuries, it can still hit you hard, for reasons that aren't always straightforward and clear.

One way of handling these fears is to discuss them with your medical team. Even if they've given you the all-clear, you might just need to hear them say the words again, or offer some specifics about why they're confident in your physical strength and stability. Feel empowered to ask for this point-blank: "I would like you to tell me why you think I'm ready to come back." Their answers alone may cause some of your anxieties and uncertainty to evaporate.

If your fears linger, don't fight them—instead, be proactive about building your confidence. The antidote to fear is confidence, a knowledge deep within your brain that you have what it takes to achieve your goals. Confidence and fear have an inverse relationship—as one rises, the other falls. Once again, it is the fuel of your thoughts and beliefs that tips the balance. If you feed your monster—the one that represents your anxieties and doubts—your fear rises while your confidence levels drop. But if you feed your confident inner athlete instead, your fear levels naturally dissipate.

There are a few specific ways of feeding your athlete that can come in particularly handy at this stage: talking yourself through it, visualizing mental strength, and using simulation training.

TALKING YOURSELF THROUGH IT

Remember, what triggers your stress response is the feeling that you can't handle the challenges in front of you. Often, your assessment of whether your abilities match up to your current demands happens subconsciously, without you even realizing it. Fortunately, you can counteract this silent inner script with a consistent, constant productive dialogue.

Coach yourself through each anxiety-producing activity not with anger and judgment, but with kindness and faith. Label your fears, normalize them, and then reassure yourself, reminding your inner athlete of all the hard work you've put in and of the objective evidence indicating that you're up to the task. You can combine this with physical cues to counteract the stress response, such as reminders to breathe and release tension.

Imagine you are talking to someone else, perhaps even a scared child, through a difficult time. Think—or actually say out loud—things like:

- "I hear you. I know you're afraid. But you've done the work in rehab. Stand tall and play strong."
- "You are stronger than ever. Your whole team knows you're ready."
- "You've got this. Keep breathing. Keep believing."

Another way to use self-talk at this stage is to redirect your focus toward the positive outcomes you want and away from the downfall you fear. If all you're thinking each time you suit up or head out is, "I don't want to get injured again," your brain has a tendency to gloss over the word "don't" and latch onto "injured." Again, at a subconscious level, you've directed your mind toward the negative emotions, thoughts, and energy associated with being sidelined.

Instead, craft a positive, facilitative script based on what you desire instead of what you fear: "I want to come back strong." "I will be mentally and physically tougher." "I want to build from the ground up and feel rock solid." Repeat these types of phrases and you'll notice your mindset subtly shift to one of calm confidence.

VISUALIZING MENTAL STRENGTH

We've discussed visualization several times—in fact, it's an essential mental skill you'll need in order to rebound. Picturing yourself performing successfully lays the groundwork for the neural pathways connecting your muscles and mind, priming you for success.

As you return to the field, game, or race course, it's especially important to conjure not only physical strength, but also mental strength. In other words, don't just see yourself performing successfully, but really *feel* it. See if you can tap into visceral emotional feelings of strength, confidence, self-assurance, skill, and calm. The Mental Movies drill at the end of the chapter offers more specific guidance on creating an effective confidence-boosting visualization script for returning to your sport.

USING SIMULATION TRAINING

Visualization can involve all your senses, but it doesn't engage your motor neurons. Simulation training goes a step further, allowing you to physically experience success in a controlled, contained environment. Much like physical rehab strengthens your body in a progressive way—with difficulty gradually increasing as you grow stronger—simulation training slowly rebuilds your confidence.

To do it, you'll create physically and emotionally safe ways to expose yourself to anxiety-producing situations—perhaps similar to those you experienced when you sustained your injury. If you need ideas, go back to the "Anxiety Pyramid" exercise on pages 113–114, and think about building from the bottom up. Your coaches and teammates are also valuable sources of ideas and assistance.

For example, say you're a cyclist who crashed on a descent. As you recover, you might place riding on a trainer at the bottom of your anxiety pyramid, while the thought of riding downhill in a pack makes you so scared you can't even imagine attempting it. First, take a deep breath, and remind yourself you don't have to jump straight there. Build up to it by starting with a short outdoor ride where it's flat, then move up the pyramid to riding downhill alone. Then recruit two or three trusted teammates to join you. You can ask them to move gradually closer to you as your anxiety about descending in a pack starts to decline.

Or, if you were injured sliding to second in a baseball game, you might start by sliding on a safer surface, then sliding into bases during practice. A more advanced simulation might involve some element of competition—for example, recruiting teammates to play a tag-like game of musical bases where only players who slide in are safe. You can practice your skills under some pressure, but without the same stakes as in an actual game. The more you build up to anxiety-producing situations and practice handling them before you reach competition, the less likely it is that they'll derail you when it truly counts.

Reconnecting mind and body

Dan Mahoney began his pro baseball career with the Jamestown Jammers, a minor-league affiliate of the Florida Marlins, based in New York. Two and a half months in—in front of a crowd larger than any he'd ever played for before—he popped his elbow throwing his first curveball. Shortly thereafter, he had Tommy John surgery to repair his ulnar collateral ligament.

Afterward, he told us in an interview, his pitching coordinator gave him two options: "'You can let the surgery define you, or you can attack it.'" Mahoney chose the latter, pushing through rehab with gusto. Each day, he'd arrive at 4:30 or 5 in the morning, often working out for an hour and a half before anyone else showed up. Nine months later, he returned to play.

His body adjusted well to his new bionic elbow. His mind, however, was a different matter. He'd always thrown with power. But now, doctors told him he had to refine his technique. His speed dropped from ninety-five to eighty-five miles per hour, and his balls weren't even close to the catcher. "It was like my identity was stripped from me after coming back because I couldn't throw hard anymore," he said.

As his struggles with the yips worsened, he began to experience anxiety and depression. The Marlins released him and Mahoney went back home to Massachusetts. He felt defeated, but knew he wasn't yet done with the game. He set about reconstructing his confidence, beginning by throwing baseballs against a brick wall at his old high school and slowly rebuilding. When the New York Yankees took a chance and signed him, he knew he needed to address his mental rehab.

So, he devoured sport psychology and mental skills books like *Thinking Body, Dancing Mind*. He realized that, for him, rebuilding his confidence required channeling some of the aggression he'd used when playing contact sports as a younger athlete. Before he took to the field, he'd fire up a heavy-metal playlist with bands like Disturbed, Five Finger Death Punch, Metallica, and Slipknot. The strategy worked, allowing him two more years in the minor leagues before he moved on.

GOODBYES, WITHOUT REGRETS

Up until now, we've placed a lot of focus on mental training in order to return to competing. But of course, the truth is that not every athlete will return. In some cases, your injury will force your hand, making it impossible for you to come back in the same capacity. In other cases, you might have a choice to make.

If you've sustained a major injury or have gone through multiple injuries, it's natural to come to a point when you ask yourself: "Do I still want to do this? Is it really worth it?" These questions grow increasingly salient as you reach the point of getting medical clearance—and they are very personal questions only you can answer. Mental skills play a key role in ensuring that *you*, and not your fears, are driving the decision.

That's why this type of work is important to do even if you are conflicted and unsure of your return. When you come back mentally strong and then make the decision to move on, you can do so without regret, on your own terms. In fact, even if you are forced to retire from your sport due to injury, mental skills work allows you to take control of your transition and move on to the next phase of your life with confidence, competence, and gratitude.

The greatest lesson of all

If every injury offers an opportunity to rebound, Alana Nichols has had more chances than most. A multisport athlete as a child, she dreamed of playing fast-pitch in the Olympics, but at the age of seventeen, she attempted a backflip on a snowboard and struck a rock, breaking three vertebrae in her back. She was paralyzed on impact.

The transition to college, adulthood, and life with a disability proved challenging, and at times so overwhelming she could barely leave her dorm room. Until one day, she rolled through the gym at the University of New Mexico and saw a team of people playing wheelchair basketball. The game was full of skill, a 24-second shot clock and regulation hoop height, even aggression as the chairs clashed. Nichols was enthralled. She got into an athletic chair that day.

Basketball swiftly became her lifeblood, what got her out of bed every day. In 2008, she went to the Paralympic Games in Beijing with the US Women's Wheelchair Basketball Team, which won gold. Soon afterward, Nichols set a new goal, and moved to Colorado to begin competing in ski racing. In 2010, she won gold medals in downhill and giant slalom in the

Winter Paralympics in Vancouver—the first woman ever to win gold in the winter and summer games.

Paralympic skiing comes with significant risks; athletes whizz down mountains with heavy equipment attached to their bodies. In June of 2013, Nichols was training at Mount Hood when she slammed feet-first into a boulder going forty miles an hour. She broke both ankles and dislocated her right shoulder.

Rehab was long and tough. She had surgery, struggled through recovery with the use of only one limb, and had difficulties withdrawing from pain medications (more on this on page 108). She began to sink down into a depression once again. This time, she was able to recognize what was happening—that her mood was low because she couldn't move her body. It still wasn't easy, but she could put it in perspective, knowing she'd feel better when she regained function.

Her body and mind still healing, she was back out on the snow by November, on a tight timeline to train for the Winter Games in Sochi the following March. She made the team and even won silver in the downhill, but then crashed during her second event, the Super G. She bounced back quickly enough to complete one more race at the Games—the giant slalom, where she came in fourth—but the whole experience sent her into a tailspin.

She contemplated retirement, especially as she considered the effects on her family of so many hospital trips, but then recommitted. "I realized I still loved this sport, to my very core, and I wasn't finished. I didn't get to leave ski racing as the person I wanted to be," she said. She decided to aim for one last Paralympic Games, PyeongChang 2018, with an entirely different mindset: "I wanted to love myself and take really good care of myself in the context of ski racing."

And she succeeded, though not in the way she'd anticipated. In February of 2018, she crashed again in a downhill ski race, sustaining cuts to her face and her seventh major concussion. Following concussion protocol meant she'd be out for a week, and the race she needed to qualify for PyeongChang was two days away. Nichols may have been able to fight her way back anyway, but chose not to. "I ultimately had to choose myself over my performance," she said. "That was the lesson, that's what I put all my energy into."

Though her career didn't conclude in exactly the way she'd expected, learning to navigate her injuries ultimately aided Nichols in moving on to her next phase. She grieved over her missed chance, but chose to watch every minute of the Olympic and Paralympic Games, publicly supporting her would-be teammates in interviews and on social media. "I decided the overarching goal of my experience as a Paralympian was to inspire others to be active and push their limits, whatever they had to do to be the best they can with what they have. My time was going to end at some point," she said. "It was really important for me to take on a new role as being a huge cheerleader."

Did you catch the rebound? Nichols bounced when she channeled her athletic energy into wheelchair basketball. She bounced again when she made peace with her transition away from ski racing and focused on the bigger picture of sport's role in her life, and her role in sport.

JUST THE FACTS

- The closer you get to medical clearance, the more anxious you may become.
- Your body may be physically primed before your mind is fully prepared to return to action.
- Setbacks are normal. Recovery isn't linear. You'll face ups and downs all along the way.
- Fear of re-injury is a normal psychological and physiological response to coming back.
- Fear of re-injury can increase your risk of getting hurt again.
- Confidence and fear have an inverse relationship—as one rises, the other falls.
- It's natural to ask yourself if you want to continue in your sport after a major injury.
- Even if injury forces you to retire or change sports, you can do so on your own terms.

MENTAL SKILLS AND DRILLS

With a continued focus on your mental skills training, you can embrace your return like Michael de Leeuw did and sync up your mental and physical readiness as Dan Mahoney did. And if it is your time to move on from your sport or into a new role within it, like Alana Nichols did, you can do so with clarity and peace. These mental drills will boost your confidence, allow you to envision success in any situation, and balance your life for the long term.

MENTAL DRILL: PERFORMANCE PROFILE 2.0

Revise your previous profile to rank yourself on the skills essential to your sport.

Mental Skills
Level 1, Rookie: Goal-Setting, Motivation
Level 2, All-Star: Self-Awareness

You first filled out a Recovery Performance Profile in Chapter 2—flip back to page 51 for a reminder and more complete instructions. As you prepare to return to your sport, revisit it so that you can reassess where you are now and start to think about creating new goals as you continue on your journey of recovery. This time, ask yourself: What are the mental and physical skills I need to excel at in order to accomplish my goals and perform in my sport? For each skill, rank yourself on a scale of 1 to 10 regarding your current ability in each skill. Recreate the chart below on a blank sheet of paper, or use the form in the workbook you can download at www.injuredathletesclub.com.

PERFORMANCE SKILL	1	2	3	4	5	6	7	8	9	10
Focus										
Communication										
Resilience										

MENTAL DRILL: ATHLETE AFFIRMATIONS

Feed your athlete with authentic and powerful self-talk.

Mental Skills
Level 1, Rookie: Confidence, Focus
Level 2, All-Star: Attitude
Level 3, Hall of Fame: Generosity, Discipline

Affirmations are positive and powerful statements uttered as if they are already true. As you prepare to return, they will prove especially powerful in boosting your confidence and reducing your fears of re-injury. When crafted and refined effectively, each statement should produce a visceral feeling of power and strength within you. As such, they're fairly personal to each athlete, but here are some examples:

- I am strong and getting stronger every day.
- I am excited to get back to competition.
- I'm mentally strong; I'm physically strong; I'm ready.
- I've prepared for this moment; I am confident and composed.

Even if you aren't quite feeling the affirmation in the moment you read it, they are reminders of what you want, and they are absolutely true.

Come up with a list of at least ten athlete affirmations. If you're having trouble, imagine the powerful and positive statements your coach, trainers, or teammates might make about you. Print out a copy of your list and post it where you'll see it every day. Take a picture of it on your phone to reference before practice. Read it regularly, and if you can, say the affirmations out loud.

MENTAL DRILL: MENTAL MOVIES

Visualize yourself performing with confidence and strength as you come back.

Mental Skills
Level 1, Rookie: Confidence, Motivation
Level 2, All-Star: Visualization

In Chapter 3, you tried out using visualization to help induce a calm mind and promote the healing of your injury—you can read more complete instructions about the technique there. Now, you're aiming to see yourself feeling strong and confident, and performing successfully. Remember, the most powerful visualization script includes all of your senses to create a vivid picture in your mind.

Start writing a script by answering the questions below:

◆ What skill or scenario would you like to see yourself perform successfully?
◆ How do you feel about that skill or scenario right now?
◆ Ideally, how would you like to feel as you execute that skill or scenario?
◆ What are some of the things you might see, hear, taste, touch, and smell during this experience?
◆ How does your body feel as it moves through space in executing this skill or scenario?

MENTAL DRILL: PLAN B

Think through stressful situations and reprogram your response in advance.

Mental Skills
Level 1, Rookie: Confidence, Focus
Level 2, All-Star: Attitude, Self-Awareness, Visualization
Level 3, Hall of Fame: Discipline, Psychological Flexibility, Resilience

When life hands us unexpected challenges and adventures, we have a tendency to *react* instead of *respond*. Your *reaction* usually comes from the more primitive parts of your brain and comprises the immediate thoughts, feelings, and behaviors that occur when you're faced with the challenging situation. Your response, meanwhile, is a thoughtful choice about how you want to handle the situation—which course of action you'll take to feel calm, confident, and in control. Responses are typically driven by your prefrontal cortex, so they can override your defensive, protective reactions.

You can't always predict what will happen during your recovery and your return to sport, but with thought, you can craft a list of possible stressful situations. Thinking through them ahead of time and considering how you'd respond—rather than how you'd react—will make it far easier to proceed in a thoughtful, productive way when each situation does arise. Use the following chart—there's a blank one in the workbook at www.injuredathletesclub.com—to come up with a list of stressful situations and considered responses. You can add oomph to this exercise by spending a few minutes visualizing each situation and then responding instead of reacting.

SITUATION (potential source of tension or stress)	REACTION (how you're likely to react initially, out of instinct)	RESPONSE (a 'Plan B' that would prove more facilitative)
Pain when you return to play	Immediately freak out, fear that you've re-injured yourself	Stop and assess whether the pain is expected or signifies a problem (using criteria you've discussed with your medical team). Based on this assessment, either continue or pull back.
An unexpected delay before you're medically cleared	Feel angry that your medical team is holding you back, have harsh words with your doctor, physical therapist, or trainer	Express your disappointment, then ask what new goals and timelines you can set to show you're ready.

MENTAL DRILL: POWER PLAYLISTS

Make lists of songs to motivate, inspire, and calm.

Mental Skills
Level 1, Rookie: Confidence, Motivation, Stress Management
Level 2, All-Star: Attitude

Research has shown that music can improve athletic performance in many ways, including by diverting your attention from fatigue, amping you up, setting your pace, and decreasing levels of the stress hormone cortisol. Start taking note of songs that make you feel calm, excited, powerful, and confident. Create a playlist for each of these moods, and listen as needed to produce those emotions.

For example, if you find yourself feeling anxious before practice, put your headphones on and listen to your Calm Power Playlist. If you're getting ready to head out to your first competition and you want to feel ready, grounded, and strong, listen to your Confidence Power Playlist. Continue adding songs and playlists as you feel inspired.

MENTAL DRILL: BALANCE THE WHEEL

Figure out your formula for a complete, happy life.

Mental Skills
Level 1, Rookie: Goal-Setting, Stress Management
Level 2, All-Star: Self-Awareness
Level 3, Hall of Fame: Discipline, Resilience

Many injured athletes struggle with a loss of their athletic identity. Who are you if you are not Brad the basketball player or Sarah the triathlete? An important part of mental-training work is to answer these questions and explore other parts of your identity.

If a cyclist brings their bike to the shop with wheel wobble, the mechanic will "true" the wheel by placing equal tension on all the spokes. Your wheel needs to be true in order to roll straight. The same applies to life; if you've put all of your "tension" and focus into your sport, leaving the rest of your life spokes loose, you may experience some "life wobble."

It's natural for you as an athlete to pour significant attention and energy into your sport. But putting energy into other parts of your life and interests creates equal tension on the spokes of the wheel, mitigating the emotional blow when part of your identity is threatened. Answering the questions below can offer you some clues to creating a better balance.

- Who are three people in your life you would like to connect with more?
- How will you connect with these people?

- What are three daily hassles you currently face
- How will you eliminate these daily hassles?

- What are three things that make you feel energized when you do them?
- How will you incorporate these things into your life?

- What are three new activities or pursuits you are interested in trying?
- How will you explore these new things?

MENTAL DRILL: THANK ME VERY MUCH

*Express your gratitude to your own body and mind for
carrying you through this process.*

Mental Skills
Level 2, All-Star: Communication
Level 3, Hall of Fame: Generosity, Psychological Flexibility

In Chapter 1 you bought yourself a sympathy card. Now it's time to express
your gratitude—to yourself. You have done an incredible job navigating a very
challenging situation. Facing an injury is one of the most stressful experiences
an athlete can endure, and you deserve some credit. Buy yourself an actual
paper card (no cheating by scribbling on a sheet of scratch paper, these symbolic
gestures carry true power).

If you have trouble carrying out this exercise, imagine writing to someone
who has been a tremendous support to you through this process. Thank
yourself for all of your hard work, for your belief during the times when it was
challenging, for continuing to move forward when you wanted to just sit down
and quit, for staying the course. Thank your body for all of its hard work, for
holding up through the process, and for working tirelessly to heal. And finally,
thank yourself for just being you.

MENTAL DRILL: GOODBYE LETTER

Use the power of the pen to help you close one chapter and open another.

Mental Skills
Level 1, Rookie: Motivation
Level 2, All-Star: Attitude, Emotional Intelligence
Level 3, Hall of Fame: Psychological Flexibility, Resilience

Whether your injury is one that has forced you to retire from your sport before
you were ready, or whether you are choosing to make that transition for yourself
and on your own terms, beginning to look at life without your sport and
redefining yourself can be distressing. This is another scenario where writing
can help you to process the many different emotions you are going through.

Write this letter as if you are writing to your best friend—but in this case, your best friend is your sport. Be sure to choose a time and a place where you will not be disturbed. Don't censor yourself as you write. Think of all the things you would want to say to someone you love.

◆ What were some of the greatest joys you experienced in your sport?
◆ What were some of your biggest losses?
◆ What were some of the greatest challenges you had to overcome?
◆ What are you grateful for?
◆ What do you feel you learned about yourself during that time?
◆ How will you continue to carry those lessons forward with you?

At the end of your letter, be sure to say goodbye. Allow yourself to grieve, and also allow yourself to look forward to the future. As with the "Write It Out" exercise in Chapter 4, it doesn't matter what you do with your letter. You can share it with your teammates, friends, and fans. You can burn it over a campfire and make s'mores. You can put it in a drawer and leave it there forever. This is your chance to honor what this time has meant to you and give yourself permission to move on.

A fond farewell

As you sit down to write your own letter, here are excerpts from the letter written by athlete Ronni Robinson, a member of the Injured Athletes Club and a freelancer writer herself.

Dear Running:
It is very painful to write this letter to you.

As you know, Running, we have been friends since I was a young child. Playing with friends and organized sports were my greatest joys.

Then, Running, we met again and got together casually in a not-forced-at-team-practice-way while I was at college. We became exclusive in the fall of 1996 when I was 28. It felt perfectly natural. I loved the fresh air, I loved seeing what my body could do, and, I'm not going to lie, I loved the calories you burned, Running.

I soon started entering road races. I did 5Ks, 10Ks, half marathons and ran a marathon. Running, we weren't super-fast and it was hard going those far distances, but I loved the structured training I followed and I loved the feeling of accomplishment when I finished.

Then in 2010, a new love entered my life—Triathlon (which means you too, Running. Please don't be mad that you were now part of a threesome).

Ooh, Triathlon, you challenged me in new ways. I had to learn to swim and I had to learn how to work the gears on a bike. There was so much to discover and so much training to do. You filled all of my needs physically, and my Type-A personality needs mentally. You were a love-at-first-sight training schedule.

Triathlon, I thought we would grow old together. But as you know, Triathlon, my left knee had other plans. Close to six years ago, the knee started to hurt. I saw the orthopedist and he ordered an MRI. I had a meniscus tear so he repaired it arthroscopically. He found I was born with a portion of the meniscus missing.

Five years later, in 2017, the knee began hurting again. Another MRI. Another tear. The arthroscope went in for the second time and cleaned up the meniscus. My recovery was a little slower this time.

In the meantime, Triathlon, you know I received an amazing gift of playing baseball at the Phillies Phantasy Camp. Early on the second day, my knee loudly told me it was unhappy with the agility moves of playing baseball. Triathlon, you know the end of that story: yet another tear to the poor, long-suffering meniscus.

The third tear was the proverbial nail in the coffin. The orthopedist didn't want to touch my knee so soon after my last surgery. The amount of cartilage under my patella had degenerated. I had a bone spur, arthritis, and a touch of tendonitis, as well. The doctor told me nothing would heal the integrity of the inside of my knee; weight-bearing activities were no longer in my future.

Triathlon, I didn't think this day would come so soon. Running, this certainly affects you the most, because swimming and biking are both low impact and easy on the knees.

Triathlon, you have been an amazing journey, which makes saying goodbye to you that much harder. You taught me how strong I was mentally. Though my training enabled me to physically endure 13-plus hours on my feet, it was my brain that kept me from quitting when the road grew rough.

Running and Triathlon, with every finish line crossed, you empowered me to feel like I could do anything to which I set my mind. I tried to pass that knowledge on to my children so they wouldn't be afraid to challenge themselves and to know they could and should reach for the stars. I was proof of that.

It is with a lost and heavy heart that I say goodbye, Running. Thank you for all the gifts you have given me in mind, body and spirit. Though I will attempt to replace you with some other activity, you will always be a tough act to follow.

CHAPTER 9

THE REBOUND LIFESTYLE

"When something traumatic happens, there's a huge surge or influx of energy, and it can go either way. You can get stuck in it or you can use it in a way that drives you forward."
—*Skier and Paralympic medalist Josh Dueck*

Just because you've returned to your sport, retired, or reached the end of this book, it doesn't mean your rebound is over. Indeed, in some cases, you may still find yourself struggling and in need of support. Fortunately, there are trained professionals who can assist—it's important to realize that it's normal to seek help, and to know where to find it. Whichever types of tools and support you use through the injury process, mental skills you've cultivated throughout your injury process can help you in other endeavors, from job interviews to health crises. Once you've learned to rebound from your injuries, each bounce can take you higher not just in your sport, but beyond it.

Wow—what a ride

"You're going to rock the world in a wheelchair."

Those words from the physician confirmed Josh Dueck's greatest fears. Dueck, a freestyle skier and coach, had overshot a trick he was showing his students and landed face-first after a 100-foot fall. Lying in the snow, he wondered why he couldn't move his legs. Now, he knew he never would again.

At the same time, the doctor's assessment gave him hope. As Dueck headed into surgery the next day, he repeated three thoughts: "Everything happens for a reason." "Nothing happens we're not strong enough to deal with." And, "Everything in my life has prepared me for this moment." (Craft your own Injury Mantras on pages 70–71.)

As he adjusted to life with paralysis, there was another bright spot. A woman he had a crush on quit her job, bought a one-way bus ticket, and stayed by his side as he began rehab. Eventually, they married.

Despite the significant challenges ahead of him, the joy of new love and the support of the community around him made it relatively easy for Dueck to primarily feel gratitude and a sense of positive forward momentum. And then there was the mindset he'd honed as an athlete and coach. He was used to setting goals and celebrating milestones along the way.

Nine months after severing his spinal cord, Dueck was back in the mountains. Sure, he had a sit ski—a bucket seat on a single ski—but the sense of freedom and connection that had drawn him to the slopes since childhood was just as strong. By the following year, he'd begun competing in ski racing. In 2010, he won a silver medal at the Paralympic Games in Vancouver.

Afterward, a downturn in his frame of mind that he called the "Paralympic hangover" set in and caught him completely off guard. Devoid of the sense of purpose that had consumed him since the first days after his accident, he fell into a deep depression. He drank more, and he lashed out at his wife Lacey and others closest to him, threatening his relationships.

Then an old friend called and asked him if he could bring his sit ski to the unmarked, unpatrolled trails of the backcountry. "It gave me some new focus and new goals and I knew that was going to be enough to pull me out of the trenches and then back into the mountains, both in the literal and [the] figurative way," Dueck said. Their adventures culminated in him becoming the first person to complete a backflip in a sit ski, an accomplishment that was documented in a web film called *The Freedom Chair*, and that earned him a guest spot on *The Ellen DeGeneres Show*. This achievement "bridged the gap" to the Games in Sochi in 2014, where he won a silver and a gold.

He knew those Games would be his last, that it was time to move on from his full-time career as an athlete. This time, he anticipated the wave of challenging emotions. Still, their depth surprised him once again. "I think the easiest way to think about that is, losing my identity of being a skier, which I've been so closely tied to for twenty-five years, is far more difficult than losing the ability of my lower body," he said.

To lift himself up, Dueck joined a therapy group. There, he worked through what he calls "emotional scar tissue"—feelings he'd never quite acknowledged from the past, that he can now reveal, observe, and release. (There's a technique to help you do this, Go FAR, on page 46.) For instance, there's the guilt he feels at the decisions he made on the day of the accident, and the fear and pain he believes he's inflicted upon others. (Read more about vicarious trauma on pages 194–195.)

But over time and with renewed intent, he's redirected the energy from those old wounds. Now, he mentors others with spinal cord injury and has partnered with the Live It! Love It! Foundation, High Fives Foundation, and Spinal Cord Injury BC to provide support for disabled outdoor adventurers and athletes. In 2016, he returned to the Paralympics in PyeongChang as a commentator and ambassador, an experience he said brought his career "full circle."

When he reflects back on his life thus far: "It's like wow, what a ride, what a trip," he said. "To have an accident such as a spinal cord injury and still go on to live a full, rewarding, fulfilling, thriving life that can be really enjoyable and also have a positive impact on a lot of people … it's a lot of gratitude, first and foremost."

Did you catch the rebound? Dueck bounced when he focused on gratitude and setting new goals after his initial injury. He bounced again when he took active steps—in the form of seeking out new adventures and clinical help—when issues like depression and guilt set in after his Paralympic competitions.

WHEN TO CALL THE PROS

We've noted from the beginning that depression and anxiety are normal components of your injury experience. However, there are times when symptoms of these conditions last longer, or strike more severely, than you can handle on your own. At this point, you may want to seek additional help to support your psychological recovery. Doing so doesn't mean you're weak or any less of an athlete. Think back to the growth mindset we discussed in Chapter 6. The strongest, smartest athletes know when to seek out experts to improve a specific component of their skills, training, or health—and psychological issues are no exception.

Consider consulting a psychologist, psychiatrist, counselor, or other mental health professional if you're nodding your head to more than one or two of the following red flags:

- Experiencing anger and confusion, frequent and swift agitation, or rapid mood swings
- Asking obsessive questions about when you'll be cleared to play
- Incurring re-injury because you've returned too soon—or delaying your comeback even though you're physically ready
- Exaggerating your progress and accomplishments, either to your trainers/coaches or to yourself
- Dwelling on minor physical complaints
- Reliving the events of your injury over and over
- Withdrawing from people in your life or social situations
- Experiencing feelings of hopelessness
- Either doing too much rehab or avoiding it completely
- Using alcohol or other drugs to self-medicate, to manage psychological distress, or to enhance performance
- Being addicted to prescribed pain medication
- Fearing weight loss or weight gain, or having symptoms of disordered eating, such as eating in secret or having an obsession with nutrition that interferes with your normal daily activities
- Having thoughts of hurting yourself, death, dying, or going away. If you find yourself contemplating suicide, call the National Suicide Prevention Lifeline at 1-800-273-8255, or chat live, online, 24/7 at suicidepreventionlifeline.org in the United States. U.K. residents, call the Samaritans on 116 123.

Again, these issues don't mean you're mentally weak or that you won't be able to return to your previous level of athletic accomplishment. Essentially, they're just signs that the challenges you're facing at the moment are greater than the resources you have available to cope with stressors and setbacks. Mental-health professionals can provide additional tools and techniques, or help you use the types of mental skills and drills outlined in this book, to enable you to come back stronger.

The following conditions and situations can also add complexity to your recovery, making it even more advisable in such circumstances to reach out to a qualified professional.

POST-TRAUMATIC STRESS DISORDER

Though some injuries come on slowly and quietly, others are a result of a crash, collision, or other catastrophic moment. Especially in those cases, athletes face a risk of post-traumatic stress disorder, or PTSD, an anxiety-based condition that develops after you witness or experience a traumatic event. PTSD often affects soldiers returning from battle, but veterans are far from the only people who experience it.

As with stress or the fear of re-injury, PTSD is physiological, representing a stress reaction that alters your brain functioning. When you have PTSD, the neurons in your brain fire differently. Levels of brain chemicals like serotonin and dopamine are altered in ways that affect your mood, reactions, and processing. Your hippocampus, which stores memories, actually shrinks. And your amygdala—which, as we described in Chapter 5, governs whether your body responds to a stimulus as stressful—becomes overly active. All this essentially short-circuits your brain to leave you in a state of heightened fear; your brain may believe you're in danger right now, rather than in the past, leading to you having intrusive thoughts about your trauma or re-living the experience. The same type of flight-or-fight response that's triggered in the face of an imminent threat occurs, even though the injury happened long ago.

Sometimes symptoms occur soon after the traumatic event, but in other cases, they may not arise until months or even years later. There are four types of symptom associated with PTSD:

- Re-experiencing the moment of your injury
- Avoiding situations that remind you of how you got hurt
- Feeling more negatively about yourself and others, including guilt, shame, or lack of interest in things you used to enjoy
- Being jittery or keyed up—a state known as "hyperarousal."

PTSD can significantly interfere with your everyday life and your return to training and competition. And it's not something you can tough your way through; often, symptoms worsen if you don't address them. The good news is that psychotherapy, medications, and other treatments work to alleviate PTSD, even if you've had it for a while. Don't be afraid to reach out if you need to. Know, too, that the same type of factors that enhance your mental recovery from injury—for instance, having coping skills and a support system—may reduce your risk of developing PTSD after a traumatic event.

Taking trauma seriously

Fiona Ford, the triathlete who crashed on her bike and who we met in Chapter 3, was a pro at applying her athletic identity and skills to her recovery—but at one point, she realized she needed to call for back-up. As she was coming off pain medications (something we touch on in Chapter 5), she reached a point where she was too sad and fearful to leave her house.

She went back to her general practitioner, who suspected PTSD and prescribed cognitive behavioral therapy, which Ford found extremely helpful. She's learned the deep impacts of trauma, and shares this message with the athletes she coaches who have been through similarly life-changing incidents.

"It doesn't just go away in a few weeks or a few months or a few years. You'll have triggers, and just as long as you know where they are and what's likely to provoke them, then you can kind of manage, with being prepared," she said. For instance, she finds it hard to watch sports like skiing on TV, when crashes are involved. After speaking about her crash at motivational events, she takes a while to recover afterward. But, with patience and time, athletes can deal with their fears in small steps and come out the other side stronger. "Often," said Ford, "extraordinary things happen if you can overcome them."

VICARIOUS TRAUMA

If you've ever felt ill when watching a teammate crash or averted your eyes from the television during the replay of a gruesome collision, you have an idea of what it's like to experience vicarious trauma. Witnessing—or in some cases, just hearing about—one of your teammates or competitors getting hurt can bring a swirl of emotions, especially if you're in the midst of recovering from your own injury. On one hand, you may feel empathetic and sad for the person who's hurt. But these events also remind you of your own fragility, leading to such emotions as fear, horror, and anxiety for yourself. Injury is a risk all athletes understand but seldom think about. When someone in your proximity falls victim to it, you have no choice but to ponder your own vulnerability.

Fear and anxiety induced by someone else's experience could, unfortunately, alter your own performance in ways that could lead to an increased risk of injury for you; while it's normal to proceed with a bit more caution after someone close to you is injured, it's important to recognize when vicarious trauma has become problematic. Many of the same tactics that can reduce your fear of re-injury also work to alleviate vicarious trauma; turn to pages 170–173 for a reminder of these. However, if vicarious trauma leads you to develop PTSD-like symptoms, you might need more support to move past it.

Understanding vicarious trauma can also shift your perspective on how your friends, family, and teammates responded to your injury. If your injury was acute and serious, you may have triggered a response of vicarious trauma in them, leading them to treat you differently or avoid you. This doesn't mean they don't care—they just may not know how to recognize or cope with their own feelings of fear and anxiety in order to be able to support you.

CONCUSSIONS

Until recent years, concussions were barely considered an injury. "Getting your bell rung" was just part of the game. You might be a little hazy or foggy, but you'd shake it off and get right back in, lest you let your team down. Today, brain imaging and other technologies have given scientists a much greater understanding of what happens to the brain during concussion, which experts also call mild traumatic brain injury (MTBI) or traumatic brain injury (TBI), depending on the severity.

Concussion occurs when an impact or sudden movement of the head—say, from a fall off your bike, a collision with another player, or a blow to your head from a ball, stick, or fist—causes your brain to move inside your skull. This impact immediately shifts levels of potassium and calcium to actually change the way electrical impulses deliver messages from neuron to neuron. Although your brain might not look any different on a CT scan or MRI, tiny structures within it may have sustained damage. This includes the axons—nerve fibers that extend from your brain cells to transmit signals.

Your brain works desperately to repair the damage and return to homeostasis, demanding significant amounts of glucose or energy—meanwhile, the blood flow to your brain is often reduced, starving your brain just when it needs fuel the most. Note that you don't actually have to lose consciousness for any of this to happen; in fact, the majority of MTBIs don't involve blacking out. The most common immediate symptoms include:

- Headaches
- Dizziness
- Confusion
- Disorientation
- Blurred vision.

Proper treatment of concussion begins with its diagnosis. Scientists are working on producing a blood or saliva test to detect concussion, but we aren't there yet. So, a neurologist or other medical professional will evaluate you using a combination of neurological testing (checking your vision, hearing, and reflexes, for instance), assessments of your thinking and memory, and sometimes brain imaging. (If you had a baseline assessment before your injury, this might be compared with your current results.) Treatment often requires complete and total rest, including avoiding any activities that involve mental effort or concentration—so, no video games, schoolwork or computer work, reading, or texting.

Most people recover completely from concussions. However, some have lingering cognitive, physical, and emotional symptoms that can last for weeks, months, or even years afterward. Doctors call this post-concussion syndrome, and symptoms include:

- Nausea
- Fatigue
- Difficulty recalling the incident
- Increased sadness
- Difficulty falling asleep
- Insomnia
- Sleeping more than usual
- Difficulty concentrating
- Jumpiness
- Irritability
- Sensitivity to light and noise
- Problems with balance
- Headaches
- Dizziness

- Anger and/or rage
- Isolation
- Fear
- Confusion
- Difficulty remembering old and/or new information.

Once you have sustained a concussion, you have an increased risk of suffering a second concussion. And if you return to your sport and receive another blow to the head before your brain is fully healed, you're also at risk of suffering from second impact syndrome—a serious condition that may result in permanent damage to the brain, a coma, or even death. In other words, concussions aren't something to be "shaken off" or taken lightly. It's critically important to seek medical attention following a head injury and to watch out for warning signs of concussion in the days, weeks, and months afterward.

Concussions can present some unique challenges when it comes to your mental recovery. First, there's the difficulty of receiving an accurate diagnosis—the symptoms can often be missed or written off, and not all physicians have specialized training in diagnosing the condition. In addition, the changes in your brain after a concussion affect your mood, motivation, and thinking. On top of that, there are the cultural influences, whereby head injuries tend to be dismissed, as well as the fact that concussion is an invisible injury, lacking any external cues for others to see why you've been sidelined. You may not even "feel" injured, making it incredibly hard to choose to stick to your recovery plan.

Whether your concussion occurs alongside other injuries or is your only injury, you'll still ride the same emotional roller coaster afterward. That makes head injuries even more psychologically complicated, since cognitive and emotional symptoms can occur both in response to injury and as a result of it. You might have symptoms of depression and anxiety from psychological causes, from neurobiological causes, or from both. You may wonder:

- Am I irritable because I'm upset about not being able to compete and just in a bad mood, or am I irritable because my brain is still healing?
- Am I sleeping more than usual because this is a symptom of depression, or am I sleeping so much because my brain is still healing?

These questions may not have simple answers, and typically require professional help to untangle. Note, too, that concussion can also interfere with your ability to complete mental drills or build your mental skills. Some of the exercises in this book might not be appropriate for you until after you've had a period of rest and recovery. Make sure to check with your neurologist or other doctor overseeing your care about how to integrate mental skills into your concussion treatment and rehab—or, if you find you aren't getting the support you need from your physicians, ask for a referral to a neuropsychologist or other health professional skilled in concussion care.

Finding—and sharing—new possibilities

At the peak of Mike Suski's boxing career in the 1980s and 90s, no one talked about concussions. Of course, Suski saw other fighters getting "punch drunk"; each time he stepped into the ring, he was petrified of a blow that would ring his bell. He knew punch-drunk fighters stood back on their heels, so he found himself constantly evaluating his form to reassure himself that he was OK. He told us in an interview that although he estimates he eventually sustained at least a dozen concussions, he—and every other fighter he knew—kept their fears and pains to themselves.

It wasn't until Suski retired and began reading medical journals that so much of his past came into perspective. He began grasping why it was that, back in 1992, after a series of hard hits from his sparring partners, he lost the motivation to fight, even though he'd earned the chance to compete in the Olympic Trials. He now had a hunch about what had really gone on in his brain when, after a nationally televised loss at the famous Palace of Auburn Hills, he went back to his dressing room with no memory of the fight, asking his dad, "When do I go up?" And ultimately, he recognized the underlying reasons for the split-second-slower reaction times and pre-fight anxiety attacks that eventually drove him out of the sport.

Afterward, he spent several years drinking and fighting—even getting a few more concussions in bar brawls. His speech was slurred, his short-term memory shot. But eventually, with the support of his then-girlfriend Michelle, he made a decision: He wasn't going to live that way anymore. In his medical fact-finding mission, he read that high-intensity exercise generates new neurons, so he began swimming as a way to boost his heart rate without impact. He quit drinking and cleaned up his diet. His cognitive abilities recovered enough that he went to college and even made the honor roll (for the first time ever).

Today, he's married to Michelle and has two kids, a gym in Mesa, Arizona, and a book, *Small Town Boxer*. He's grateful for the adventurous life boxing offered him and for the turnaround he's experienced. But as he sees former elites and pros in contact sports struggling or even contemplating or dying by suicide, he's determined to alert athletes—especially young ones—to the emotional fallout concussions can cause. If they know now what he didn't know back then, he believes, they might at least have hope that better days lie ahead.

UNCERTAIN DIAGNOSES

As we noted back in Chapter 2, humans typically don't cope well with uncertainty. When you develop pain or can't function at your best as an athlete, your first instinct is to hunt for answers: Why is this happening? How can I fix it? How long until I'm back to training and competing?

In some cases, injured athletes receive definitive explanations. An MRI shows a clear stress fracture, doctors can identify a torn ligament, a joint is visibly dislocated. Medical professionals can draw on scientific studies, as well as on their experience treating a given injury, to describe your likely path forward. But in other cases, even the brightest medical minds and most advanced imaging technology can't pinpoint the exact cause of your problems.

There's no doubt that these situations are incredibly frustrating. You might find yourself wishing for a diagnosis—any diagnosis, including the worst one— just so you have an understanding of what's happening to you. However, even if some of the steps toward physical recovery remain unclear, mental skills can help you navigate your psychological recovery. If you keep your focus on the present moment, harness your support system to navigate the medical system, practice holding conflicting beliefs at the same time, and prioritize relaxation and self-care, you may find yourself already on the rebound, despite the lack of a definitive diagnosis.

Some mental drills that may help you navigate this process include:

◆ Go FAR (Chapter 2)
◆ Bad News/Good News (Chapter 2)
◆ Stop/Start/Continue (Chapter 3)
◆ In/Out of Control (Chapter 4)

- Mindfulness Meditation (Chapter 4)
- R&R (Chapter 5)
- Stress Busters (Chapter 5)
- Build Your Team (Chapter 6)

You may also want to revisit the advice on seeking second opinions in Chapter 6.

Thriving through doubts

Nicole Mericle ran competitively in high school, then in college at Rice University; her main event was the steeplechase. During her fifth year there, in 2011, she tore the labrum in her left hip. The summer between her fourth and fifth years, she developed an interest in climbing. "At the time, though, my [running] coach said—no climbing," she told us. "I listened to him."

After several rounds of physical therapy—as well as narrowly averting surgery—Mericle had reduced the pain in her hip enough to pursue a post-collegiate running career. By then, she'd moved to Boulder, where both running and climbing were possible. Though she was a swift learner in climbing, progressing quickly to master a 5.12c-grade route, she focused on running. She joined an elite team and eventually worked her way back up to sixty-mile weeks.

Soon, though, she began developing a strange sensation in her right leg, a feeling that she couldn't control it. This baffling injury plagued her on and off, and she bounced from appointment to appointment, consulted nerve specialists, underwent 3D gait analyses, but no one was able to give her an answer.

By the fall of 2016, she still lacked a diagnosis, and grew tired of seeking one. "I had to basically make a decision that I wasn't going to try to run on roads or flat ground; I was going to give up on my dream of running the steeplechase again or running fast on roads," she said. "It really did feel like giving up for a long time. I kind of had to reframe my mentality to think, 'OK, it's really just shifting my goals. It's OK to accept that something may not be perfect again, but you do your best with the body that you have.'"

Even as she hung up her track spikes, Mericle noticed something. When she took her run off-road—to hills, to trails—she didn't feel the same symptoms. So, only wanting to run enough to be a "happy human," that's what she did. Little by little, without any expectations, she improved. Eventually, she realized she might be able to compete in trail running. She hired a coach to guide her. This time, she chose one who understood that climbing also played a large role in her happiness, and who would support her in pursuing two types of training that were sometimes at odds. She also hired a climbing coach to keep that part of her training on track.

Though it's not always smooth sailing, she's exploited her strengths and combined her passions in a thriving career as an obstacle course racer. In 2016, her first year in the sport, she came in second at the Obstacle Course Racing World Championships in the 15K. In 2018, she won the 3K at the OCR World Championships; by April 2019, she was ranked the top in the world in the sport.

HOW TO FIND AN EXPERT

The mental skills and drills in this book will give you a head start on addressing your psychological recovery alongside your physical rehab. But if you have the warning signs listed at the beginning of the chapter, if you continue to struggle with feelings of depression or anxiety, if you have difficulties fully accepting and adjusting to your injured status, if you are contemplating a transition out of sport, or if you just need someone in your corner you can trust as a sounding board to help support you through this journey, you might want to find a qualified practitioner to assist you.

The decision as to whether to seek out psychotherapeutic support or mental skills training (or both) depends on your goals, your level of distress, and whether you are experiencing a diagnosable mental or emotional disorder or simply want education and skills to enhance your performance. With both options you want to be sure you are working with a qualified professional who has been specially trained in the services you need.

SPORT PSYCHOLOGISTS

These professionals are trained in clinical psychology as well as having specific education and expertise in the sport sciences. They are licensed psychologists who can provide psychological services and interventions for clinical issues that can arise for athletes, including:

◆ Eating disorders
◆ Substance abuse
◆ PTSD
◆ Clinical anxiety and depression
◆ Clinical depression
◆ Suicidal thoughts or behaviors
◆ Overtraining and burnout
◆ Aggression and violence
◆ Transitions out of sport.

CERTIFIED MENTAL PERFORMANCE CONSULTANTS (CMPC)

Often referred to as mental skills coaches or certified performance enhancement consultants, these qualified and trained professionals work with teams and individuals on mental skills training to enhance performance. They do not work with diagnosable mental disorders, so if these issues arise, the athlete is referred to a sport psychologist or other mental health professional for support and treatment. Sometimes mental skills coaches or performance enhancement consultants will also have another certification or licensure—they may be, for example, a licensed marriage and family therapist (LMFT)—but if you're focusing on returning from athletic injury, you're going to want someone who also has their CMPC.

Mental skills coaches or mental performance consultants help you:

◆ Build confidence
◆ Perform under pressure
◆ Hone your skills of concentration
◆ Manage performance anxiety
◆ Understand effective goal-setting principles
◆ Learn mindfulness and relaxation skills
◆ Develop stress-management and coping skills.

If you're looking for support in these areas, you can find qualified professionals through one of these organizations:

◆ Association for Applied Sport Psychology (AASP)
www.appliedsportpsych.org
◆ The British Association of Sport and Exercise Sciences (BASES)
www.bases.org.uk

If you're in school, check with your athletic department or school counseling office regarding available resources. Of course, pro and elite teams often have these types of consultants on staff. And no matter what level you play or compete at, you can always ask for a referral from a friend, teammate, coach, physician, or athletic trainer.

BEYOND SPORT

This injury probably isn't the first hardship you have encountered, and you can bet it won't be the last. You'll undoubtedly face other painful challenges in life and will be amazed at your own strength once you get to the other side. When you approach your injury in the way outlined in this book, you'll find the lessons it teaches you apply to so many other difficult moments in life.

One of the most amazing things about dedicating yourself to working on your mental fitness during your injury recovery is that *these mental skills remain powerful post-injury as well*. Consider this work an investment in yourself—a time of studying, taking inventory, acknowledging your strengths, and examining the places where growth is needed. Mental skills represent the knowledge and tools you need to support that growth, to move from wishing for positive outcomes to actually bringing them about. Take one more look at the list of mental skills you've worked on through these pages:

◆ Confidence
◆ Focus
◆ Goal-setting
◆ Motivation
◆ Stress management
◆ Attitude
◆ Communication
◆ Emotional intelligence
◆ Self-awareness
◆ Visualization
◆ Discipline

◆ Generosity
◆ Mindfulness
◆ Psychological flexibility
◆ Resilience.

Consider what you could accomplish if you were armed with all these abilities. These aren't just injury-recovery skills—these are life skills. We can't think of a single situation you'll encounter where these proficiencies won't serve you. Committing to yourself and recognizing that your mental recovery is just as important as your physical recovery builds an ever-expanding toolkit of techniques to cope with any challenge life throws your way, from other health setbacks to relationship and financial troubles to personal losses.

There's a myth we all too frequently buy into when it comes to happiness—that all the joy, peace, satisfaction, and contentment we seek awaits us just around the corner. Happiness, we're told, will arrive at a specific point in the future when everything falls magically into place. But then, when we reach that distant point, something else comes up and robs us of our rightful bliss.

Eventually, we have to come to terms with the fact that we are the ones stealing our own happiness. Though it's difficult to grasp, once this news sinks in, you can view it as a liberation. You don't have to wait to be happy, you can claim what you deserve right here and right now. Joy and peace come from accepting the lows as well as the highs. If you hone your mental skills, each impact point becomes an opportunity to bounce back higher. What's more, the transitions between setbacks and victories no longer feel like waiting periods to endure or rush through, but significant and essential pieces of a bigger picture. Even when everything is in flux and you don't know exactly what's in store for you, you can feel confident in your ability to handle just about anything.

Coming back from an injury really can be an opportunity to start again—to begin with a fresh slate and build yourself up the way you want to. Don't just think about getting back to the athlete you were, consider the person you want to become. Back in Chapter 3 on pages 74–75 we asked you to write your injury story as a hero's journey. Reflect on that journey now—flip back to that exercise if you need to jog your memory. How are you better for having gone through this experience? How can you build up from this new knowledge? Returning to competition from injury, or even retiring from your sport, might mark the end of a chapter—but each of us is writing a full book. As one journey concludes, you're just on the cusp of a new one. How will you step into your role?

Forging new identities

For a while, 2010 ranked as the most difficult year in Jillion Potter's life. That was the year she broke her neck, after all. But that was only the first of several challenges to come.

First, though, the injury. During a game in Canada, the then-captain of the US women's rugby team found herself at the bottom of a tangle known in rugby as a ruck. She felt her neck pop, and worried. But she was able to walk off the field to the sidelines, from where she watched the rest of the game, and then rode to the hospital in her trainer's car. She didn't find out she'd broken a vertebra and ruptured a disc until three weeks later. Doctors operated on her—using bones from her hip to fuse her cracked spine together—and told her she'd never play again.

Though her friends, parents, and some of her doctors might have preferred otherwise, Potter fought back and returned to play less than a year later. She moved to Denver and joined a club team, unsure if she'd choose to climb back to the sport's highest levels. Then she got wind of an inaugural American team in rugby sevens, a version of the sport with fewer players and a shorter time-clock than rugby union, which she'd been playing since college. Soon, she was invited to move to San Diego and join that team.

They won a bronze medal in the 2013 Rugby World Cup Sevens in Moscow, and Potter suddenly had a new goal: in 2016, women's rugby—in the form of sevens—would be part of the Olympics for the first time ever. As one of the country's dominant players, little would stand in her way of making it to Rio. Until, that is, August 2014, when doctors removed a 10x8x3-centimeter tumor from her jaw and told her she had stage 3 synovial sarcoma, a rare and often fatal cancer.

Potter's diagnosis added a new dimension to her goal: it now became beating cancer so that she could get to Rio. To get there, she started literally one step at a time, she told us. "During treatment, my wife and I would walk every day before my infusion. It would take me forever to walk around the block, but I was determined to do it, because it was going to get me to the Olympics."

During her off days from chemo, Potter worked out so hard she passed out. She drank the highest-calorie supplements she could find to combat the weight loss that started during her infusions and continued through radiation. Eight weeks after she completed treatment, she ran a half marathon. A year later, she was named to the first-ever American Olympic women's sevens team, which wound up placing fifth.

Unfortunately, Potter's cancer returned five months later. This time, she realized, she couldn't count on the momentum of an international sporting competition to pull her through. So she used other coping strategies. She leaned on her support team, anchored by her wife, Carol Fabrizio. She demanded physical therapy, even though she wasn't aiming to get back to immediate training, to combat weak muscles and sore joints from treatment. She walked her dogs, got acupuncture, meditated daily, and built a backyard fence. Friends visited to do yoga or share a cup of coffee; roasting her own beans is another passion. (Make a start on nurturing your passions with the Balance the Wheel drill on page 183.)

And above all, she tried to stay grateful. "My life is awesome. Even when I had cancer, my life was awesome. You know I still had a great wife, great home, I had wonderful friends, I had awesome days. Did I wish I didn't have cancer? Absolutely, but I wouldn't trade any of those moments of the good days."

She was declared cancer-free in February 2018. Now, Potter has new goals. She's aiming to go back to the Olympics—this time as a referee, a process she calls humbling. "As a player you think, 'Yeah, I know the law, I know how to play.' But as a ref, it is like ten times harder." And she has lingering effects from her treatments that hamper her, including a speech impediment from surgery that left her tongue numb.

Still, she's determined, and not just because she craves a new physical test. She thrives on players' gratitude at having an Olympian among them, and hopes she serves as an example of how to have a fulfilling life in sport beyond competition. It's the same reason she'll respond to any fans or players who reach out to her in person or on social media.

One message she gives them: The physical training required to overcome obstacles and compete at a high level is significant, but so too is the mental piece of the puzzle. Her speed, and her confidence as a player, shifted after cancer, but that didn't stop her from becoming an Olympian—or from thriving once the Games were behind her.

> "You have to acknowledge that you've changed physically, emotionally, all those things, and then don't hold on too tightly to the past and what you used to be," she said. "You almost have to selectively forget that identity that you had, because you are creating a new one. You've changed. And that's a hard thing to do, but I think acknowledging that is very much a part of overcoming injury or illness and getting back to sports, or life."

Did you catch the rebound? Potter bounced when she supported her team during her injury. She bounced again when she made the choice to train for Rio despite her cancer diagnosis—and again when she approached the process differently the second time around.

Did you catch YOUR rebound? As you've worked your way through this book and read other athletes' stories, we hope you've also been able to spot the times YOU bounced during your injury journey. We'd encourage you to write these down and celebrate them.

JUST THE FACTS

- You are not weak, you are not alone, and you are still an athlete.
- If you're privileged enough to call yourself an athlete for long enough, you will probably face injury at some point along the way.
- Injuries cause a roller coaster of emotions, many of them negative, but you won't always feel this way.
- Many athletes have overcome serious life-altering injuries to make what experts call remarkable recoveries—dramatic physical and psychological comebacks.
- Everyone's recovery process looks different. Focus on *your* progress and *your* goals.
- Try not to look at things only under a microscope. Your injury is part of a bigger picture.
- Mental skills give you incredible power to overcome obstacles and bounce back stronger—to rebound.
- You will get through this. You might even realize, eventually, that you're better for it.

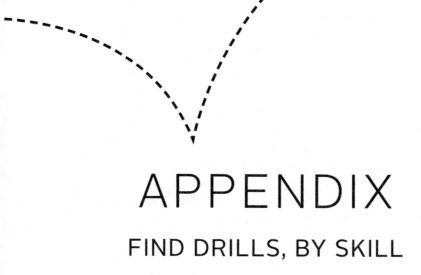

APPENDIX

FIND DRILLS, BY SKILL

Do you have an idea of where you'd like to focus your mental skills work? Here, you will find all the exercises that relate to each of the fifteen key mental skills essential to the rebound.

Level 1—Rookie

SKILL	DEFINITION	DRILLS
Confidence	Belief and trust in your ability to accomplish your goals.	Sidelined SWOT; Redefine Success; Grab Your Goals; Healing Visions; Yes, And...; Random Reminders; Anxiety Pyramid; Build Your Team; Chart Your Confidence; Flip the Script; Seeing is Believing; Compare with Compassion; Athlete Affirmations; Mental Movies; Plan B; Power Playlists

SKILL	DEFINITION	DRILLS
Focus	Capacity to direct or redirect your energy and attention to what's relevant and constructive.	Go FAR; Obstacles to Opportunities; Bad News/Good News; Stop/Start/Continue; Grab Your Goals; Time-Travel Log; In/Out of Control; Feel and Focus; Mindfulness Meditation; Energy Conservation; Pain Log; Stress Busters; Found in Translation; Chart Your Confidence; Thoughtstopper; Seeing is Believing; Athlete Affirmations; Plan B
Goal-Setting	Ability to define what you want to accomplish and create a plan to achieve that target.	Recovery Performance Profile; Stop/Start/Continue; Grab Your Goals; Anxiety Pyramid; Can You Cope?; Build Your Team; Flip the Script; Performance Profile 2.0; Balance the Wheel
Motivation	Drive and desire to put in the work and push toward your goals and aspirations.	Sidelined SWOT; Recovery Performance Profile; Stop/Start/Continue; Grab Your Goals; Hero's Journey; Feel and Focus; Random Reminders; Build Your Team; Join the Club; Chart Your Confidence; Seeing is Believing; Performance Profile 2.0; Mental Movies; Power Playlists; Goodbye Letter
Stress Management	Proficiency at using coping skills and strategies to eliminate stressors when you can and to regulate the stress response when you can't.	Emotion Decoder; Laugh Out Loud; Go FAR; Injury Mantras; In/Out of Control; Mindfulness Meditation; Energy Conservation; Random Reminders; Write It Out; R&R; Anxiety Pyramid; Can You Cope?; Stress Busters; Build Your Team; Join the Club; Give Thanks; Flip the Script; Thoughtstopper; Seeing is Believing; Compare with Compassion; Pen Pals; Power Playlists; Balance the Wheel

Level 2—All-Star

SKILL	DEFINITION	DRILLS
Attitude	Positive approach and mindset to facing adversity, challenges, and setbacks.	Go FAR; Obstacles to Opportunities; Good News/Bad News; Funhouse Mirror; Redefine Success; Injury Mantras; Hero's Journey; Yes, And...; Feel and Focus; Random Reminders; Write It Out; Here's What's Up, Doc; Found in Translation; Give Thanks; Flip the Script; Compare with Compassion; Athlete Affirmations; Plan B; Power Playlists; Goodbye Letter

SKILL	DEFINITION	DRILLS
Communication	Competence at clearly expressing your opinions and ideas—and ability to hear and understand others' perspectives.	My Condolences; Yes, And...; Pain Log; Build Your Team; Here's What's Up, Doc; Found in Translation; Communication Cheat Sheet; Give Thanks; Flip the Script; Pen Pals; Thank Me Very Much
Emotional Intelligence	Ability to recognize emotions, discern their origins, and understand how they affect behavior.	Emotion Decoder; My Condolences; Go FAR; Good News/Bad News; Funhouse Mirror; Feel and Focus; Write It Out; Found in Translation; Flip the Script; Thoughtstopper; Goodbye Letter
Self-Awareness	Conscious knowledge about how you operate, including how you think, feel, and react.	Emotion Decoder; Injury Intake Form; Sidelined SWOT; Laugh Out Loud; Go FAR; Funhouse Mirror; Recovery Performance Profile; Stop/Start/Continue; Time-Travel Log; Feel and Focus; Pain Log; Anxiety Pyramid; Can You Cope?; Stress Busters; Build Your Team; Here's What's Up, Doc; Communication Cheat Sheet; Chart Your Confidence; Performance Profile 2.0; Plan B; Balance the Wheel
Visualization	Skillfulness at creating and recreating vivid, controllable images in your mind.	Healing Visions; Energy Conservation; R&R; Anxiety Pyramid; Thoughtstopper; Seeing is Believing; Mental Movies; Plan B

Level 3—Hall of Fame

SKILL	DEFINITION	DRILLS
Discipline	Persistence in pursuit of longer-term goals and deeper values.	Sidelined SWOT; Obstacles to Opportunities; Stop/Start/Continue; Grab Your Goals; In/Out of Control; R&R; Here's What's Up, Doc; Found in Translation; Communication Cheat Sheet; Compare with Compassion; Athlete Affirmations; Plan B; Balance the Wheel

SKILL	DEFINITION	DRILLS
Generosity	Willingness to extend grace toward yourself and others.	My Condolences; Laugh Out Loud; Go FAR; Redefine Success; Injury Mantras; Hero's Journey; Yes, And...; Random Reminders; Stress Busters; Build Your Team; Join the Club; Here's What's Up, Doc; Found in Translation; Communication Cheat Sheet; Give Thanks; Compare with Compassion; Athlete Affirmations; Thank Me Very Much
Mindfulness	Adeptness at keeping your consciousness in the present moment— or at bringing it back there—and acting as an objective observer of your own experience.	Go FAR; Healing Visions; Time-Travel Log; In/Out of Control; Feel and Focus; Mindfulness Meditation; Energy Conservation; R&R
Psychological Flexibility	Willingness and ability to adapt to changing circumstances by shifting your reactions, behaviors, and perspective.	Go FAR; Obstacles to Opportunities; Good News/Bad News; Funhouse Mirror; Redefine Success; Hero's Journey; Yes, And...; Write It Out; Found in Translation; Communication Cheat Sheet; Pen Pals; Plan B; Thank Me Very Much; Goodbye Letter
Resilience	Power to bounce back from hardship or adversity and thrive despite setbacks.	Laugh Out Loud; Go FAR; Obstacles to Opportunities; Injury Mantras; Hero's Journey; Feel and Focus; Random Reminders; Can You Cope?; Stress Busters; Chart Your Confidence; Plan B; Balance the Wheel; Goodbye Letter

MENTAL DRILLS

These are the mental drills that address the greatest number of mental skills—in other words, if you're only going to focus on a few, they'll give you the biggest bang for your buck.

- Go FAR
- Feel and Focus
- Anxiety Pyramid
- Build Your Team
- Found in Translation
- Flip the Script
- Plan B.

ACKNOWLEDGMENTS

CINDY AND CARRIE SAY ...

We're incredibly indebted to all the currently or previously injured athletes we interviewed for this book. We know it's not always easy to discuss the most difficult parts of your journeys, but we were struck by your openness and generosity, and your willingness to help others by participating. Thanks also to the thoughtful and knowledgeable experts we've consulted along the way—your input was invaluable. We'd also like to thank our editors at Bloomsbury, Matthew Lowing and Zoë Blanc, for believing in this project and for their expert guidance. Finally, gratitude to Matt Kuzma for allowing us to take over our house as a workspace, and Megan Imundo for compiling our resources.

CARRIE SAYS ...

I still remember, many years ago, sitting in my very first class in graduate school studying sport psychology and thinking to myself, "This is crazy. Why don't more people know about this?" It wasn't until college that I really came into my athletic life, and in non-traditional sports like car racing, snowboarding, and rock climbing. Before I made my way to graduate school I didn't know sport psychology existed, which means that when I sustained my first major injury, a torn meniscus, I didn't have the benefit of any mental recovery.

Fast forward a few years and by chance, I ended up injuring that same knee (this time a torn MCL) during my graduate studies in sport psychology. As soon as it happened, I decided I would use all the knowledge I was acquiring to help athletes build confidence, mental toughness, and resilience, and apply it to my own injury recovery. The difference in my recovery from my first knee injury to my second was profound, and that's barely a strong enough word for it. Honestly, I was shocked. Therefore, the first thing I want to acknowledge is how grateful I am for my injury experiences. Without them, I wouldn't have found my way to writing this book.

The second acknowledgment I have is the gratitude I feel for all of the injured athletes I have spoken to and consulted with in my professional work. More than anything, it was you that inspired this book. I am indebted to all of you for opening up, sharing your stories, and trusting me to help in your recovery. It is such a gift and I learned so much from each and every one of you. And I'd especially like to thank my collaborator on this project, Cindy Kuzma. I'd originally set out to do this as a solo endeavor, and I'm SO glad I didn't. Thank you for all of your support, your hours of effort, and your tireless help throughout this project. And thanks for saying yes to a perfect stranger when she invited you to spend a week with her in Asheville! And to my family and friends for their continued support and patience while I disappeared from my family and social life so I could dedicate time to write this book. You guys are the best and I'm so blessed to have you on my "crew."

CINDY SAYS ...

Four stress fractures, high hamstring tendinopathy, Achilles problems—my medical resume already more than qualified me to work on a book about coping with injury. When I developed another foot problem while training for the Boston Marathon in 2018—and in the middle of completing the first draft—I developed an entirely new appreciation for the power of mental rehab. When, at the last minute, my diagnosis changed and I was able to run the race after weeks off of training, I drew on so many of the tactics I learned from Carrie to make it through. Injury is never ideal, but I'm grateful to have had that experience at that time as a reminder of the emotional impact—and a powerful demonstration that her methods truly work.

I can't thank Carrie enough for that, and for bringing all her tremendous professional expertise to this project; for essentially allowing me to invite myself to her book retreat in Asheville; and for trusting that we could, together, do work that truly helps people overcome significant setbacks. To all my running partners, coaches, and the mutual cheering squad of athletes I'm lucky enough to know—I so appreciate everyone who's discussed their struggles, asked me questions, and listened to me breathlessly discuss how much I learned from, and believed in, this work. I'm also grateful to my current and former editors at *Runner's World* and other outlets who have allowed me to explore these topics in print and online, including but certainly not limited to Sarah Lorge Butler, Katie Neitz, Meghan Kita, Brian Dalek, and Christa Sgobba. Members of my writing group in Chicago—Claire Zulkey, Dawn Reiss, Kelly James, and Megy Karydes—were invaluable sources of support and feedback. Thanks also to my parents, Bill and Mary Szelag—who always believe in me and have still saved the first-ever book I wrote—and my equally supportive in-laws, Matt and Charlene (and Lucas) Kuzma. And most of all, to Matt, for all the things. You're still the best decision I've made, and I don't know where I'd be without your support.

ABOUT THE
AUTHORS

Carrie Jackson Cheadle lives in Northern California and is a Mental Skills Coach and Certified Mental Performance Consultant through the Association for Applied Sport Psychology. She is author of the book *On Top of Your Game: Mental Skills to Maximize Your Athletic Performance* (Feed the Athlete Press, 2013). A popular source for media, Carrie has been interviewed for numerous publications, including *Men's Fitness, Women's Health, Outside Magazine, Shape Magazine, Runner's World, Bicycling Magazine,* and the *Huffington Post.*

Carrie received her bachelor's degree in psychology at Sonoma State University, California, and her master's degree in sport psychology at John F. Kennedy University, California. She has been teaching and supervising master's students in the Sport Psychology program at that same university since 2006. She consults with athletes of all ages and at every level, from recreational athletes to high school and collegiate athletes, to elite and professional athletes competing at national and international levels. In addition to being known for her expertise in sports performance and psychological recovery from injury, she is one of the foremost experts specializing in mental skills training for athletes and exercisers with Type 1 diabetes, and is the director of the Mental Skills Training Program for Diabetes Training Camp. Carrie has her own personal commitment to lifelong fitness, and when she isn't working with athletes, you might find her running on a trail, playing guitar, or hitting the slopes on her snowboard.

Cindy Kuzma is a Chicago-based journalist with a specialty in fitness and health. Her work has appeared in such publications as *Runner's World*, *The New York Times*, *Chicago Magazine*, *Men's Health*, *Women's Health*, *espnW.com*, VICE's *Tonic*, *SELF*, *OutsideOnline.com*, *Prevention*, *USA Today*, and elsewhere. She also contributed audio reporting to the podcasts *The Runner's World Show* and *Human Race*, produced by *Runner's World*, and co-hosts #WeGotGoals, a podcast by Chicago-based media company aSweatLife.com. She's completed more than twenty marathons, including seven Boston Marathons, and also likes to lift heavy things. She studied journalism at Baylor University and has a master's degree from Northwestern University's Medill School of Journalism, along with additional coursework in anatomy, physiology, and biology. She lives in the Andersonville neighborhood with her husband and two cats/interns, Mushaboom and Tuna.

Together, Cindy and Carrie are administrators of The Injured Athletes Club on Facebook and co-hosts of The Injured Athletes Club podcast.

InjuredAthletesClub.com
carriecheadle.com
cindykuzma.com

REFERENCES

INTRODUCTION

"2018 Boston Marathon results" http://registration.baa.org/2018/cf/public/iframe_Results Search.cfm?mode=results [accessed September 2018].

"Allie Kieffer: America's next great distance runner" https://www.fleetfeet.com/blog/allie-kieffer-americas-next-great-distance-runner [accessed September 2018].

Ardern, C. L., Taylor, N. F., Feller, J. A., and Webster, K. E. (2013) "A systematic review of the psychological factors associated with returning to sport following injury," *British Journal of Sports Medicine*, 47(17): 1120–1126.

Arvinen-Barrow, M., Clement, D., Hamson-Utley, J. J., Zakrajsek, R. A., Lee, S. M., Kamphoff, C., Lintunen, T., Hemmings, B., and Martin, S. B. (2015) "Athletes' use of mental skills during sport injury rehabilitation," *Journal of Sport Rehabilitation*, 24(2): 189–197.

Brees, D. and Fabry, C. (2011) *Coming Back Stronger: Unleashing the Hidden Power of Adversity* (Carol Stream, IL: Tyndale House Publishers).

Fendrich, H. (2018) "Broken bones, torn ligaments , more: Lindsey Vonn's injuries" http://www.aspentimes.com/pyeongchang-2018-winter-olympics/broken-bones-torn-ligaments-more-lindsey-vonns-injuries [accessed April 2019].

Grant, T. (2018) "The effect of psychological response on recovery of sport injury: A review of the literature," *Kinesiology, Sport Studies, and Physical Education Synthesis Projects*, 45 Volume or page number?.

Hall, S. (@sarahall3). (2019) Photograph of Sara Hall and accompanying caption, dated 12 January. https://www.instagram.com/p/Bsih72UFHDL.

Kieffer, A. (@kiefferallie). (2019) Photograph of Allie Kieffer and accompanying caption, dated March 21. https://wwww.instagram.com/p/BvSUlfvAtTX.

Kriebel, A. "Olympic Skier Lindsey Vonn Shares How Strength, Determination, and Self-Love Have Propelled Her to the Finish Line." http://www.ourbodybook.com/

olympic-skier-lindsey-vonn-shares-how-strength-determination-and-self-love-have-propelled-her-to-the-finish-line [accessed April 2019]

Multhaupt, G., and Beuth, J. (2018) "The use of imagery in athletic injury rehabilitation: A systematic review," *German Journal of Sports Medicine*, 69: 57–64.

Paine, N. (2018) "Lindsey Vonn Is The Greatest American Skier — And It's Not Even Close," https://fivethirtyeight.com/features/lindsey-vonn-is-the-greatest-american-skier-and-its-not-even-close [accessed April 2019].

Salim, J., Wadey, R., and Diss, C. (2016) "Examining hardiness, coping and stress-related growth following sport injury," *Journal of Applied Sport Psychology*, 28: 154–169.

Sherman R. (2019) "The Case for Drew Brees As the Quarterback GOAT," http://www.theringer.com/nfl/2018/10/9/17956106/drew-brees-career-passing-yards-record-qb-greatness [accessed April 2019].

Sonesson, S., Kvist, J., Ardern, C., Österberg, A., and Silbernagel, K. G. (2017) "Psychological factors are important to return to pre-injury sport activity after anterior cruciate ligament reconstruction: Expect and motivate to satisfy," *Knee Surgery, Sports Traumatology, Arthroscopy*, 25: 1375–1384.

Tatsumi, T., and Takenouchi, T. (2014) "Causal relationships between the psychological acceptance process of athletic injury and athletic rehabilitation behavior," *Journal of Physical Therapy Science*, 26(4): 1247–1257.

CHAPTER 1

Allen, H. (2019) "Progress is Not Perfection." https://hillygoat.wordpress.com/2019/02/02/progress-is-not-perfection [accessed April 2019].

Appaneal, R. N., Levine, B. R., Perna, F. M., and Roh, J. L. (2009) "Measuring postinjury depression among male and female competitive athletes," *Journal of Sport and Exercise Psychology*, 31: 60–76.

Ardern, C. L., Taylor, N. F., Feller, J. A., and Webster, K. E. (2013) "A systematic review of the psychological factors associated with returning to sport following injury," *British Journal of Sports Medicine*, 47: 1120–1126.

Birkett, D. (2018) "Detroit Lions' Brandon Copeland dangerous, determined in comeback" https://www.freep.com/story/sports/nfl/lions/2018/02/13/detroit–lions–brandon–copeland/332661002/ [accessed August 2018].

Bunch, E. (2017) "How Allie Kieffer pushed past her fitness breaking point to place 5th at the NYC marathon" https://www.wellandgood.com/good–sweat/allie–kieffer–fitness–running–advice/ [accessed September 2018].

Chung, Y. (2012) "Psychological correlates of athletic injuries: Hardiness, life stress, and cognitive appraisal," *International Journal of Applied Sports Sciences*, 24(2): 89–98.

Day, M. C., Bond, K., and Smith, B. (2013) "Holding it together: Coping with vicarious trauma in sport," *Psychology of Sport and Exercise*, 14: 1–11.

"Fuel performance review: Michael Neal" https://www.indyfuelhockey.com/news/detail/fuel–performance–review–michael–neal [accessed August 2018].

Johnson, G. (2018) "New York Jets sign Penn alum" https://penntoday.upenn.edu/news/new–york–jets–sign–penn–alum [accessed September 2018].

Kuzma, C. (2016) "Alia Gray's Chicago hope" https://www.runnersworld.com/news/a20824854/alia–grays–chicago–hope/ [accessed September 2018].

Lamont-Mills, A., and Christensen, S. A. (2006) "Athletic identity and its relationship to sport participation levels," *Journal of Science and Medicine in Sport*, 9: 472–478.

Leddy, M. H., Lambert, M. J., and Ogles, B. M. (1994) "Psychological consequences of athletic injury among high-level competitors," *Research Quarterly for Exercise and Sport*, 65(4): 347–354.

Lichtenstein, M. B., Gudex, C., Andersen, K., Bojesen, A. B., and Jørgensen, U. (2017) "Do exercisers with musculoskeletal injuries report symptoms of depression and stress?" *Journal of Sport Rehabilitation*, 1–6.

Madrigal, L. (2014) "Psychological responses of Division I female athletes throughout injury recovery: A case study approach," *Journal of Clinical Sport Psychology*, 8: 276–298.

National Suicide Prevention Lifeline https://suicidepreventionlifeline.org/ [accessed August 2018].

Neal, T. (2015) "Recognizing the signs" https://athleticmanagement.com/2013/08/17/recognizing_the_signs/index.php [accessed August 2018].

Polloreno, J. B. (2018) "Hillary Allen's triumphant return to ultrarunning" https://womensrunning.competitor.com/2018/07/inspiration/hillary–allens–triumphant–return–to–ultrarunning_96904 [accessed August 2018].

"Psychological issues related to illness and injury in athletes and the team physician: A consensus statement—2016 update," *Current Sports Medicine Reports*, 16(3): 189–201.

Reese, L. M. S., Pittsinger, R., and Yang, J. (2012) "Effectiveness of psychological intervention following sport injury," *Journal of Sport and Health Science*, 1: 71–79.

Salim, J., and Wadey, R. (2018). "Can emotional disclosure promote sport injury-related growth?" *Journal of Applied Sport Psychology*, 30(4): 367–387.

Steele, R. (2015) "Penn football's Brandon Copeland continues to chase NFL dream," https://www.thedp.com/article/2015/08/former–penn–football–linebacker–brandon–copeland–shot–detroit–lions–performance–app [accessed August 2018].

Stypulkoski, M. (2018) "How a lost season converted Jets' Brandon Copeland from NFL outcast to key contributor," https://www.nj.com/jets/index.ssf/2018/08/how_a_lost_season_propelled_jets_brandon_copeland.html [accessed September 2018].

Tatsumi, T., and Takenouchi, T. (2014) "Causal relationships between the psychological acceptance process of athletic injury and athletic rehabilitation behavior," *Journal of Physical Therapy Science*, 26(4): 1247–1257.

"The 41st Annual Utica Boilermaker 15k Road Race" http://leonetiming.com/2018/Roads/Boilermaker/15kGunTime.htm [accessed September 2018].

Tracey, J. (2003) "The emotional response to the injury and rehabilitation process," *Journal of Applied Sport Psychology*, 15: 279–293.

US Paralympics (2017) "U.S. Powerlifters Claim Silver Medal and Record Five Additional Top-15 Finishes at World Championships," https://www.teamusa.org/US–Paralympics/Features/2017/December/12/US–powerlifters–claim–silver–medal–and–record–five–additional–top–15–finishes–at–world–championships [accessed September 2018].

CHAPTER 2

Chödrön, P. (2012) *Living Beautifully: With uncertainty and change* (Boulder, CO: Shambhala).

Hamson-Utley, J. J., and Vazquez, L. (2008) "The comeback: Rehabilitating the psychological injury," *Sport Psychology & Counseling*, 13(5): 35–38.

Huysmans, Z., and Clement, D. (2017) "A preliminary exploration of the application of self-compassion within the context of sport injury," *Journal of Sport & Exercise Psychology*, 39: 56–66.

Lewis, M. (2016) "Why we're hardwired to hate uncertainty" https://www.theguardian.com/commentisfree/2016/apr/04/uncertainty–stressful–research–neuroscience [accessed March 2018].

Neff, K. D., Kirkpatrick, K. L., and Rude, S. S. (2007) "Self-compassion and adaptive psychological functioning," *Journal of Research in Personality*, 41: 139–154.

Salim, J., Wadey, R., and Diss, C. (2016) "Examining hardiness, coping and stress-related growth following sport injury," *Journal of Applied Sport Psychology*, 28: 154–169.

Savage, J., Collins, D., and Cruickshank, A. (2017) "Exploring traumas in the development of talent: What are they, what do they do, and what do they require?" *Journal of Applied Sport Psychology*, 29: 101–117.

Wadey, R., Evans, L., Hanton, S., and Neil, R. (2012) "An examination of hardiness throughout the sport injury process," *British Journal of Health Psychology*, 17: 103–128.

Wadey, R., Podlog, L., Galli, N., and Mellalieu, S. D. (2016) "Stress-related growth following sport injury: Examining the applicability of the organismic valuing theory," *Scandinavian Journal of Medicine & Science in Sports*, 26: 1132–1139.

CHAPTER 3

Arvinen-Barrow, M., Clement, D., Hamson-Utley, J. J., Zakrajsek, R. A., Lee, S. -M., Kamphoff, C., Lintunen, T., Hemmings, B., and Martin, S. B. (2015) "Athletes' use of mental skills during sport injury rehabilitation," *Journal of Sport Rehabilitation*, 24: 189–197.

Creasy, J. W., Rearick, M. P., Buriak, J., and Motley, K. R. (2012) "Indicators of rehabilitation noncompliance among college athletics: A review of the literature," *Athletic Training and Sports Health Care*, 4(2): 94–96.

Grindley, E. J., Zizzi, S. J., and Nasypany, A. M. (2008) "Use of Protection Motivation Theory, affect, and barriers to understand and predict adherence to outpatient rehabilitation," *Physical Therapy*, 88(12): 1529–1540.

Heil, J., Wakefield, C., and Reed, C. (1998) "Patient as athlete: A metaphor for injury rehabilitation," *The Psychotherapy Patient*, 10(3–4): 21–39.

Ironman World Championship 2007 official results http://www.ironman.com/assets/files/results/worldchampionship/2007.pdf [accessed May 2018].

Kappes, A., Singmann, H., and Oettingen, G. (2012) "Mental contrasting instigates goal pursuit by linking obstacles of reality with instrumental behavior," *Journal of Experimental Social Psychology*, 48: 811–818.

Lengacher, C. A., Bennett, M. P., Gonzalez, L., Gilvary, D., Cox, C. E., Cantor, A., Jacobsen, P. B., Yang, C., and Djeu, J. (2008) "Immune responses to guided imagery during breast cancer treatment," *Biological Research for Nursing*, 9(3): 205–214.

Maddison, R., Prapavessis, H., Clatworthy, M., Hall, C., Foley, L., Harper, T., Cupal, D., and Brewer, B. (2012) "Guided imagery to improve functional outcomes post-anterior cruciate ligament repair: Randomized-controlled pilot trial," *Scandinavian Journal of Medicine & Science in Sports*, 22: 816–821.

Robinson, A. (2015) "About," https://www.alirobinsonracing.com/about.html [accessed June 2018].

Robinson, A. (2015) "Triathlon results 2015," https://www.alirobinsonracing.com/results.html [accessed June 2018].

Taylor, A. H., and May, S. (1996) "Threat and coping appraisal as determinants of compliance with sports injury rehabilitation: An application of Protection Motivation Theory," *Journal of Sports Sciences*, 14: 471–482.

Wiese-Bjornstal, D. M., Smith, A. M., Shaffer, S. M., and Morrey, M. A. (1998) "An integrated model of response to sport injury: Psychological and sociological dynamics," *Journal of Applied Sport Psychology*, 10(1): 46–69.

CHAPTER 4

"'All I could think of was her': Catherine Tyree's turning point," https://heelsdownmag.com/all–i–could–think–of–was–her–catherine–tyrees–turning–point/ [accessed June 2018].

"Altra Golden Ticket Races," https://www.wser.org/golden–ticket–races/ [accessed July 2018].

Bennett, J., and Lindsay, P. (2016) "Case study 3: An acceptance commitment and mindfulness based intervention for a female hockey player experiencing post injury performance anxiety," *Sport and Exercise Psychology Review*, 12(2): 36–45.

Boone, A. (2016) "2016: A year of healing," http://www.ameliabooneracing.com/blog/rehab/2016-a-year-of-healing [accessed August 2018].

Boone, A. (2016) "Finding joy in the DNS," http://www.ameliabooneracing.com/blog/rehab/finding-joy-in-the-dns [accessed August 2018].

Boone, A. (2016) "Recovery: On realizing you aren't superhuman," http://www.ameliabooneracing.com/blog/uncategorized/superhuman [accessed August 2018].

Boone, A. (2016) "When it all comes crashing down," http://www.ameliabooneracing.com/blog/uncategorized/injury-when-it-all-comes-crashing-down [accessed August 2018].

Boone, A. (2016) "'When will you be back?'" http://www.ameliabooneracing.com/blog/worldstoughestmudder/when-will-you-be-back [accessed August 2018].

Boone, A. (2018) "2017: A year of rediscovering joy," http://www.ameliabooneracing.com/blog/spartan/2017-year-rediscovering-joy [accessed September 2018].

Boone, A. (2019) "Don't Fight the Water," http://www.ameliabooneracing.com/blog/uncategorized/dontfightthewater [accessed August 2019]

Chamberlin, J. (2008) "The time of our lives," *Monitor on Psychology*, 39(9): 20 http://www.apa.org/monitor/2008/10/time.aspx [accessed May 2018].

Dalek, B. (2018) "When the course wins: No finishers at the 2018 Barkley Marathons," https://www.runnersworld.com/news/a20866366/no-finishers-at-2018-barkley-marathons [accessed August 2018].

"David Wise," https://usskiandsnowboard.org/athletes/david-wise [accessed July 2018].

Glavan, A. (2016) "Free style VH Polderhof dies in ring at WEF," http://www.chronofhorse.com/article/free-style-vh-polderhof-dies-ring-wef [accessed July 2018].

Hayes, S. C., and Wilson, K. G. (1994) "Acceptance and commitment therapy: Altering the verbal support for experiential avoidance," *The Behavior Analyst*, 17(2): 289–303.

Kashdan, T. B., and Rottenberg, J. (2010) "Psychological flexibility as a fundamental aspect of health," *Clinical Psychology Review*, 30(7): 865–878.

Mahoney, J., and Hanrahan, S. J. (2011) "A brief educational intervention using acceptance and commitment therapy: Four injured athletes' experiences," *Journal of Clinical Sport Psychology*, 5: 252–273.

"Meditation: In depth," https://nccih.nih.gov/health/meditation/overview.htm [accessed September 2018].

"Mindfulness exercises," https://www.mayoclinic.org/healthy-lifestyle/consumer-health/in-depth/mindfulness-exercises/art-20046356 [accessed September 2018].

Moore, Z. E. (2009) "Theoretical and empirical developments of the Mindfulness–Acceptance–Commitment (MAC) approach to performance enhancement," *Journal of Clinical Sports Psychology*, 4: 291–302.

Morin, A. (2017) "How to stop worrying about things you can't change," https://www.psychologytoday.com/us/blog/what-mentally-strong-people-dont-do/201705/how-stop-worrying-about-things-you-cant-change [accessed July 2018].

Murray, C. (2018) "After two adversity-filled years, David Wise back on top of game ahead of Olympic run" https://www.rgj.com/story/sports/college/nevada/2018/02/16/after-two-adversity-filled-years-david-wise-back-top-game-ahead-olympic-run/345057002 [accessed July 2018].

Nicely, J. (2017) "Jennifer Nicely: About," https://jennifernicely.squarespace.com/about [accessed July 2018].

Nicely, J. (2017) "Jennifer Nicely: On coming back from a nearly career-ending injury," https://www.climbing.com/people/jennifer-nicely-coming-back-from-a-nearly-career-ending-injury [accessed June 2018].

Perry, S. K. (2009) "Do you live in the past, present, or future?" https://www.psychologytoday.com/us/blog/creating-in-flow/200908/do-you-live-in-the-past-present-or-future [accessed July 2018].

Pisarczyk, M. (2017). "Back in the saddle," http://apps.northbynorthwestern.com/magazine/2017/winter/quad/in-saddle [accessed June 2018].

"Sean O'Brien 2016 – 100k results" https://livensr.com/sob16/results.100k.php [accessed July 2018].

Stephenson, M. (2018) "Amelia Boone is stronger than ever," https://www.runnersworld.com/runners-stories/a20652405/amelia-boone-is-stronger-than-ever [accessed July 2018].

Sword, R. K. M., and Zimbardo, P. (2016) "The importance of our time perspective," https://www.psychologytoday.com/us/blog/the-time-cure/201607/the-importance-our-time-perspective [accessed July 2018].

"Tough Mudder: Obstacles," https://toughmudder.com/obstacles [accessed July 2018].

"Western States 100-Mile Endurance Run," https://www.wser.org/ [accessed July 2018].

Wise, D. (2018) "My road to PyeongChang," https://mrdavidwise.com/my-road-to-pyeongchang [accessed July 2018].

"World's Toughest Mudder," https://toughmudder.com/events/2018-worlds-toughest-mudder [accessed July 2018].

CHAPTER 5

"About—Adam Whiting Yoga," http://www.adamwhitingyoga.com/about/ [accessed September 2018].

Albinson, C. B., and Petrie, T. A. (2003) "Cognitive appraisals, stress, and coping: Preinjury and postinjury factors influencing psychological adjustment to sport injury," *Journal of Sport Rehabilitation*, 12: 306–322.

Dutch, T. (2017) "Jordan Hasay's Boston Marathon debut was for her mother," https://www.flotrack.org/articles/5064069-jordan-hasays-boston-marathon-debut-was-for-her-mother [accessed August 2018].

Fisher, J. (2018) "5 top American women to watch: Boston Marathon 2018," https://patch.com/massachusetts/boston/5-top-american-women-watch-boston-marathon-2018 [accessed August 2018].

Garland, E. L. (2012) "Pain processing in the human nervous system: A selective review of nocioceptive and biobehavioral pathways," *Primary Care*, 39(3): 561–571.

Gilbert, J. N., Lyon, H., and Wahl, M.-t. (2015) "Coping with the stress of athletic injury: How coaches can help," *Strategies*, 28(4): 33–39.

Hainline, B., Derman, W., Vernec, A., Budgett, R., Deie, M., Dvořák, Harle, C., Herring, S.A., McNamee, M., Meeuwisse, W., Moseley, G.L., Omololu, B., Orchard, J., Pipe, A., Pluim, B.M., Ræder, Siebert, C., Stewart, M., Stuart, M., Turner, J.A., Ware, M., Zideman, D., and Engebretsen, L. (2017) "International Olympic Committee consensus statement on pain management in elite athletes," *British Journal of Sports Medicine*, 51: 1245–1258.

Heil, J. (2012) "Pain on the run: Injury, pain and performance in a distance runner," *The Sport Psychologist*, 26: 540–550.

Ivarsson, A., Johnson, U., Andersen, M. B., Tranaeus, U., Stenling, A., and Lindwall, M. (2017) "Psychosocial factors and sport injuries: Meta-analyses for prediction and prevention," *Sports Medicine*, 47: 353–365.

Johnson, U., and Ivarsson, A. (2011) "Psychological predictors of sport injuries among junior soccer players," *Scandinavian Journal of Medicine and Science in Sports*, 21(1): 129–136.

Laux, P., Krumm, B., Diers, M., and Flor, H. (2015) "Recovery–stress balance and injury risk in professional football players: A prospective study," *Journal of Sports Sciences*, 33(20) 2140–2148.

Lorge Butler, S. (2018) "Jordan Hasay Discusses the Devastating Injury That Forced Her to Withdraw From Chicago," https://www.runnersworld.com/news/a23322818/jordan-hasay-withdraw-from-chicago-marathon [accessed September 2018].

Lorge Butler, S. (2019) " After Third at Boston, Full Speed Ahead for Jordan Hasay," https://www.runnersworld.com/news/a27045776/jordan-hasay-boston-marathon-2019 [accessed April 2019].

Lorge Butler, S. (2019) " Older, Wiser, Stronger: Jordan Hasay Heads to Boston Healthy," https://www.runnersworld.com/news/a27086411/jordan-hasay-heads-to-boston healthy [accessed April 2019].

Low, P. (2017) "Overview of the autonomic nervous system," https://www.merckmanuals.com/home/brain,-spinal-cord,-and-nerve-disorders/autonomic-nervous-system-disorders/overview-of-the-autonomic-nervous-system [accessed August 2018].

Maddison, R., and Prapavessis, H. (2005) "A psychological approach to the prediction and prevention of athletic injury," *Journal of Sport and Exercise Psychology*, 27: 289–310.

"Managing pain with medications after orthopaedic surgery," http://orthoinfo.aaos.org/en/recovery/managing-pain-with-medications [accessed August 2018].

Mitchell, I. (2011) "Social support and psychological responses in sport-injury rehabilitation," *Sport and Exercise Psychology Review*, 7(2): 30–44.

"Parasympathetic nervous system," https://www.ncbi.nlm.nih.gov/pubmedhealth/PMHT0025459 [accessed August 2018].

"Progressive Muscle Relaxation for Stress and Insomnia," https://www.webmd.com/sleep-disorders/muscle-relaxation-for-stress-insomnia [accessed September 2018].

Roos, M. (2018) "Jordan Hasay drops out of the 2018 Boston marathon," https://www.womensrunning.com/2018/04/boston2018/jordan-hasay-drops-2018-boston-marathon_91588 [accessed August 2018].

Salwin, E., and Zając, A. (2016) "Pain tolerance in sport," *Baltic Journal of Health and Physical Activity*, 8(3): 71–80.

Stout, E. (2017) "Jordan Hasay calls on memory of her mom during her first marathon," https://www.runnersworld.com/news/a20853394/jordan-hasay-calls-on-memory-of-her-mom-during-her-first-marathon [accessed August 2018].

"Stress effects on the body," http://www.apa.org/helpcenter/stress-body.aspx [accessed August 2018].

"Understanding the stress response," https://www.health.harvard.edu/staying-healthy/understanding-the-stress-response [accessed August 2018].

Zach, S., Dobersek, U., Filho, E., Inglis, V., and Tenenbaum, G. (2018) "A meta-analysis of mental imagery effects on post-injury functional mobility, perceived pain, and self-efficacy," *Psychology of Sport and Exercise*, 34: 79–87.

CHAPTER 6

Benson, J. (2018) "I broke my leg; this was my recovery," http://www.therightfits.com/2018/06/i-broke-my-leg-this-was-my-recovery [accessed July 2018].

Clement, D., Hamson-Utley, J., Arvinen-Barrow, M., Kamphoff, C., Zakrajsek, R. A., and Martin, S. B. (2012) "College athletes' expectations about injury rehabilitation with an athletic trainer," *Athletic Therapy and Training*, 17(4): 18–25.

Clement, D., and Shannon, V.R. (2011) "Injured athletes' perceptions about social support," *Journal of Sport Rehabilitation*, 20: 457–470.

"CrossFit Games: About the games," https://games.crossfit.com/about-the-games [accessed July 2018].

Dweck, C. (2006) *Mindset: The New Psychology of Success* (New York: Random House).

Gilbert, J. N., Lyon, H., and Wahl, M.-t. (2015) "Coping with the stress of athletic injury: How coaches can help," *Strategies*, 28(4): 33–39.

Kampf, J. (2016) "Crossfit Games: Healthy Scott Panchik eyes championship," http://news-herald.com/20160718/crossfit-games-healthy-scott-panchik-eyes-championship [accessed July 2018].

Kuzma, C. (2018) "Have to miss your destination race? Get some money back," http://runnersworld.com/races-places/a20707855/have-to-miss-your-destination-race-get-some-money-back [accessed July 2018].

Lu, F. J. H., and Hsu, Y. (2013) "Injured athletes' rehabilitation beliefs and subjective well-being: The contribution of hope and social support," *Journal of Athletic Training*, 48(1): 92–98.

Mitchell, I. (2011) "Social support and psychological responses in sport-injury rehabilitation," *Sport and Exercise Psychology Review*, 7(2): 30–44.

Mitchell, I., Evans, L., Rees, T., and Hardy, L. (2014) "Stressors, social support, and tests of the buffering hypothesis: Effects on psychological responses of injured athletes," *British Journal of Health Psychology*, 19: 486–508.

Myers, N. L., and Capilouto, G. J. (2016) "A model for rehabilitation adherence in athletes demonstrating different attachment styles," *Human Kinetics—International Journal of Athletic Therapy and Training*, 21(4): 12–17.

Salim, J., and Wadey, R. (2018) "Can emotional disclosure promote sport injury-related growth?" *Journal of Applied Sport Psychology*, 30(4): 367–387.

"Scott Panchik," https://games.crossfit.com/athlete/34796 [accessed July 2018].

Sieff, J., and Bunch, J. (2012) "Overcoming adversity: Scott Panchik," https://games.crossfit.com/article/overcoming-adversity-scott-panchik [accessed July 2018].

Wittkamp, A. (2016) "The Crossfit Open, explained," https://games.crossfit.com/article/crossfit-open-explained [accessed July 2018].

Yang, J., Schaefer, J. T., Zhang, N., Covassin, T., Ding, K., and Heiden, E. (2014) "Social support from the athletic trainer and symptoms of depression and anxiety at return to play," *Journal of Athletic Training*, 49(6): 773–779.

CHAPTER 7

Birk, J. L., Rogers, A. H., Shahane, A. D., and Urry, H. L. (2018) "The heart of control: Proactive cognitive control training limits anxious cardiac arousal under stress," *Motivation and Emotion*, 42: 64–78.

Durden, M. (2017) "Utilizing imagery to enhance injury rehabilitation," *Sport Journal*, 1.

Hanson, S. J., McCullagh, P., and Tonymon, P. (1992) "The relationship of personality characteristics, life stress, and coping resources to athletic injury," *Journal of Sport and Exercise Psychology*, 14(3): 262–272.

Lieberman, M. D., Eisenberger, N. I., Crockett, M. J., Tom, S. M., Pfeifer, J. H., and Way, B. M. (2007) "Putting feelings into words: Affect labeling disrupts amygdala activity in response to affective stimuli," *Psychological Science*, 18(5): 421–428.

Lofthouse, G. (2015) "How language influences emotion," https://www.theatlantic.com/health/archive/2015/12/the-book-of-human-emotions-language-feelings/420978 [accessed August 2018].

Lu, F. J. H., and Hsu, Y. (2013) "Injured athletes' rehabilitation beliefs and subjective well-being: The contribution of hope and social support," *Journal of Athletic Training*, 48(1) 92–98.

Ochsner, K. N., and Gross, J. J. (2005) "The cognitive control of emotion," *TRENDS in Cognitive Sciences*, 9(5): 242–249.

Parkerson, E., Harris, B., Langdon, J., and Czech, D. (2015) "Using a motivational general-mastery imagery to improve the self-efficacy of youth gymnasts." *Journal of Applied Sport Psychology*, 26(1), 66-81.

Syed, M. (2018) *You Are Awesome: Find your confidence and dare to be brilliant at (almost) anything* (London: Wren & Rook).

Wadey, R., Evans, L., Hanton, S., and Neil, R. (2012) "An examination of hardiness throughout the sport-injury process: A qualitative follow-up study," *British Journal of Health Psychology*, 17: 872–893.

Wesch, N., Hall, C., Prapavessis, H., Maddison, R., Bassett, S., Foley, L., Brooks, S., and Forwell, L. (2012) "Self-efficacy, imagery use, and adherence during injury rehabilitation," *Scandinavian Journal of Medicine and Science in Sports*, 22: 695–703.

Zangerl, B. (2018) "Into the Void," *Rock and Ice*, 249 Volume or page number?.

CHAPTER 8

Andrew, N., Wolfe, R., Cameron, P., Richardson, M., Page, R., Bucknill, A., and Gabbe, B. (2014) "The impact of sport and active recreation injuries on physical activity at 12 months post-injury," *Scandinavian Journal of Medicine and Science in Sports*, 24: 377–385.

Ardern, C. L., Taylor, N. F., Feller, J. A., and Webster, K. E. (2012) "Fear of re-injury in people who have returned to sport following anterior cruciate ligament reconstruction surgery," *Journal of Science and Medicine in Sport*, 15: 488–495.

Basic, A. (2018) "Michael de Leeuw is coming back. How does he fit in the current Fire squad?" https://www.hottimeinoldtown.com/2018/7/26/17619142/cf97-chicago-fire-michael-de-leeuw-injury-return-how-to-fit [accessed September 2018].

Chicago Fire Communications. (2017) "Michael de Leeuw undergoes reconstructive surgery to repair a ruptured left anterior-cruciate ligament," https://www.chicago-fire.com/post/2017/11/09/michael-de-leeuw-undergoes-reconstructive-surgery-repair-ruptured-left-anterior [accessed September 2018].

Covassin, T., McAllister-Deitrick, J., Bleecker, A., Heiden, E. O., and Yang, J. (2015) "Examining time-loss and fear of re-injury in athletes," *Journal of Sport Behavior*, 38(4): 394–403.

Evans, L., Hardy, L., and Fleming, S. (2000) "Intervention strategies with injured athletes: An action research study," *The Sport Psychologist*, 14: 188–206.

Floyd, T. (2017) "Fire playmaker De Leeuw sidelined by torn ACL," http://www.goal.com/en-us/news/mls-news-chicago-fire-playmaker-michael-de-leeuw-sidelined/1m77h6njy5bh918smis9w4vr78 [accessed September 2018].

Huang, C.A., and Lynch, J. (1994) *Thinking Body, Dancing Mind: Taosports for extraordinary performance in athletics, business, and life* (New York: Bantam Books).

Johnston, L. H., and Carroll, D. (2000) "The psychological impact of injury: Effects of prior sport and exercise involvement," *British Journal of Sports Medicine*, 34: 436–439.

Krause, K. (2014) "Game to teach softball players how to slide," https://fastpitchlane.softballsuccess.com/2014/02/06/game-to-teach-softball-players-how-to-slide [accessed September 2018].

Mahoney, D. (2016) "Bio: Mahoney Performance Training," http://mahoneyperformancetraining.com/bio [accessed September 2018].

Podlog, L., Dimmock, J., and Miller, J. (2011) "A review of return to sport concerns following injury rehabilitation: Practitioner strategies for enhancing recovery outcomes," *Physical Therapy in Sport*, 12: 36–42.

Podlog, L., Lochbaum, M., and Stevens, T. (2010) "Need satisfaction, well-being, and perceived return-to-sport outcomes among injured athletes," *Journal of Applied Sport Psychology*, 22: 167–182.

Proctor, M. "Sliding fundamentals for baseball players," https://www.active.com/baseball/articles/sliding-fundamentals-for-baseball-players [accessed September 2018].

Santaromita, D. (2017) "Why Fire's draw against New York City FC could be a sign of things to come," https://www.nbcsports.com/chicago/chicago-fire/why-fires-draw-against-new-york-city-fc-could-be-sign-things-come [accessed September 2018].

Santaromita, D. (2017) "Worst-case scenario: Michael de Leeuw out for season with ACL rupture," https://www.nbcsports.com/chicago/fire/worst-case-scenario-michael-de-leeuw-out-season-acl-rupture [accessed September 2018].

CHAPTER 9

"About USA Rugby," https://www.usarugby.org/about-usa-rugby/ [accessed September 2018].

Anderson, L. (2016) "U.S. Rugby 7s "enforcer" Jillion Potter is the only help you'd need in a rumble," https://bleacherreport.com/articles/2654564-us-rugby-7s-enforcer-jillion-potter-is-the-only-help-youd-need-in-a-rumble [accessed September 2018].

Bloom, G. A., Horton, A. S., McCrory, P., and Johnston, K. M. (2004) "Sport psychology and concussion: New impacts to explore," *British Journal of Sports Medicine*, 38(5): 519–521.

Bohn, K. (2017) "Molecules in spit may be able to diagnose and predict length of concussions," https://news.psu.edu/story/495094/2017/11/20/research/molecules-spit-may-be-able-diagnose-and-predict-length-concussions [accessed September 2018].

Borg, C., Tham, D., and Stewart, A. (2016) "Jillion Potter: U.S. rugby survivor targets Olympic glory in Rio," https://www-m.cnn.com/2016/07/07/sport/jillion-potter-usa-womens-rugby-olympic-games-rio-2016/index.html?r=https%3A%2F%2Fwww.google.com%2F [accessed September 2018].

Chertok, G. J. (2013) "Psychological aspects of concussion recovery," *Sport Psychology and Counseling*, 18(3): 7–9.

"Concussion: Diagnosis & treatment," https://www.mayoclinic.org/diseases-conditions/concussion/diagnosis-treatment/drc-20355600 [accessed September 2018].

"Concussion: Symptoms and causes," https://www.mayoclinic.org/diseases-conditions/concussion/symptoms-causes/syc-20355594 [accessed September 2018].

Davies, S. C., and Bird, B. M. (2015) "Motivations for underreporting suspected concussion in college athletics," *Journal of Clinical Sport Psychology*, 9: 101–115.

Day, M. C., Bond, K., and Smith, B. (2013) "Holding it together: Coping with vicarious trauma in sport," *Psychology of Sport and Exercise*, 14: 1–11.

"Dealing with trauma: Recovering from frightening events," https://newsinhealth.nih.gov/2018/06/dealing-trauma [accessed September 2018].

Dunfee, R. (2012) "Returning to risk: The how and why," https://www.powder.com/stories/returning-to-risk-the-how-and-why/ [accessed September 2018].

"Facts about concussion and brain injury," https://www.cdc.gov/headsup/pdfs/providers/facts_about_concussion_tbi-a.pdf [accessed September 2018].

Giza, C. C., and Hovda, D. A. (2014) "The new neurometabolic cascade of concussion," *Neurosurgery*, 75: S24–S33.

Grose, J. (2016) "The Lenny Interview: USA Rugby captain Jillion Potter," https://www.lennyletter.com/story/the-lenny-interview-usa-rugby-captain-jillion-potter [accessed September 2018].

Herzog, T., and Hays, K. F. (2012) "Therapist or mental skills coach? How to decide," *The Sports Psychologist*, 26: 486–499.

Ivarsson, A., Stambulova, N., and Johnson, U. (2018) "Injury as a career transition: Experiences of a Swedish elite handball player," *International Journal of Sport and Exercise Psychology*, 16(4): 365–381.

"Josh Dueck" http://paralympic.ca/josh-dueck [accessed September 2018].

Kellmann, M., Bertollo, M., Bosquet, L., Brink, M., Coutts, A. J., Duffield, R., Erlacher, D., Halson, S. L., Hecksteden, A., Heidari, J., Kallus, K. W., Meeusen, R., Mujika, I., Robazza, C., Skorski, S., Venter, R., and Beckmann, J. (2018) "Recovery and performance in sport: Consensus statement," *International Journal of Sports Physiology and Performance*, 13: 240–245.

Kontos, A. P., Collins, M., and Russo, S. A. (2004) "An introduction to sports concussion for the sport psychology consultant," *Journal of Applied Sport Psychology*, 16: 220–235.

Kraus, N., Thompson, E. C., Krizman, J., Cook, K., White-Schwoch, T., and LaBella, C. R. (2016) "Auditory biological marker of concussion in children," *Scientific Reports*, 6.

Meeusen, R., Duclos, M., Gleeson, M., Rietjens, G., Steinacker, J., and Urhausen, A. (2006) "Prevention, diagnosis and treatment of the Overtraining Syndrome," *European Journal of Sport Science*, 6(1): 1–14.

Meyer, J. (2016) "Surviving a broken neck and cancer, Jillion Potter becomes an Olympian and part of history" https://www.denverpost.com/2016/08/07/jillion-potter-us-womens-rugby-olympics-cancer-broken-neck/?productCode=WebAccessSP [accessed September 2018].

Meyer, J. (2017) "Denver's Jillion Potter facing a second bout with cancer five months after becoming an Olympian in Rio," https://www.denverpost.com/2017/01/19/olympian-jillion-potter-facing-cancer-again [accessed September 2018].

National Center for PTSD. (2018) "Understanding PTSD and PTSD treatment," https://www.ptsd.va.gov/public/understanding_ptsd/booklet.pdf [accessed September 2018].

O'Neill, D. F. (2008) "Injury contagion in alpine ski racing: The effect of injury on teammates," performance," *Journal of Clinical Sport Psychology*, 2: 278–292.

Saffary, R., Chin, L. S., and Cantu, R. C. (2012) "From concussion to chronic traumatic encephalopathy: A review," *Journal of Clinical Sport Psychology*, 6: 351–362.

Shearer, D. A., Mellalieu, S. D., and Shearer, C. R. (2011) "Posttraumatic stress disorder: A case study of an elite rifle shooter," *Journal of Clinical Sport Psychology*, 5: 134–147.

Sherin, J.E., and Nemeroff, C.B. (2011) "Post-traumatic stress disorder: The neurobiological impact of psychological trauma," *Dialogues in Clinical Neuroscience*, 13(3): 263–278.

Smith, A. M., and Milliner, E. K. (1994) "Injured athletes and the risk of suicide," *Journal of Athletic Training*, 29(4): 337–341.

"Sport psychology," http://www.apa.org/ed/graduate/specialize/sports.aspx [accessed September 2018].

Stifter, J. (2011). "Backstory: 'The Freedom Chair,'" https://www.powder.com/stories/backstory-the-freedom-chair [accessed September 2018].

Suski, M. (2017) *Small Town Boxer* (Austin, TX: Next Century Publishing).

"What is PTSD?" https://www.ptsd.va.gov/public/PTSD-overview/basics/what-is-ptsd.asp [accessed September 2018].

Wiese-Bjornstal, D. M., White, A. C., Russell, H. C., and Smith, A. M. (2015) "Psychology of sport concussions," *Kinesiology Review*, 4: 169–189.

OTHER RESEARCH

Brewer, B. W., and Redmond, C. J. (2016) *Psychology of Sport Injury* (Champaign, IL: Human Kinetics).

Catalano, E. M., and Hardin, K. N. (1996) *The Chronic Pain Control Workbook: A step-by-step guide for coping with and overcoming pain*, 2nd edition (Oakland, CA: New Harbinger Publications).

Cheadle, C. (2013) *On Top of Your Game: Mental skills to maximize your athletic performance* (Petaluma, CA: Feed the Athlete Press).

Chödrön, P. (2016) *When Things Fall Apart: Heart advice for difficult times* (Boulder, CO: Shambhala).

Clement, D., Arvinen-Barrow, M., and Fetty, T. (2015) "Psychosocial responses during different phases of sport-injury rehabilitation: A qualitative study," *Journal of Athletic Training*, 50(1): 95–104.

Clement, D., Shannon, V. R., and Connole, I. J. (2012) "Performance enhancement groups for injured athletes, part 1: Preparation and development," *Sport Psychology and Counseling*, 17(3): 34–36.

Clement, D., Shannon, V. R, and Connole, I. J. (2012) "Performance enhancement groups for injured athletes, part 2: Implementation and facilitation," *Sport Psychology and Counseling*, 17(5): 38–40.

Crossman, J. (2001) *Coping with Sports Injuries: Psychological strategies for rehabilitation* (New York: Oxford University Press).

Crowe, K., and McDowell, E. (2017) *There is No Good Card for This: What to say and do when life is scary, awful, and unfair to people you love* (San Francisco: HarperOne).

Davis, M., Eshelman, E. R., and McKay, M. (2008) *The Relaxation and Stress Reduction Workbook*, 6th edition (Oakland, CA: New Harbinger Publications).

Gayman, A. M., and Crossman, J. (2003) "A qualitative analysis of how the timing of the onset of sports injuries influences athlete reactions," *Journal of Sport Behavior*, 26(3): 255–272.

Goleman, D. (2005) *Emotional Intelligence: Why it can matter more than IQ* (New York: Bantam Books).

Granito, V. J., Jr. (2001) "Athletic injury experience: A qualitative focus group approach," *Journal of Sport Behavior*, 24(1): 63–83.

Granito, V. J., Jr., Hogan, J. B., and Varnum, L. K. (1995) "The performance enhancement group program: Integrating sport psychology and rehabilitation," *Journal of Athletic Training*, 30(4): 328–331.

Hamson-Utley, J. J., and Vazquez, L. (2008) "The comeback: Rehabilitating the psychological injury," *Sport Psychology and Counseling*, 13(5): 35–38.

Heil, J. (1995) *Psychology of Sport Injury* (Champaign, IL: Human Kinetics).

Koch, R. (1999) *The 80/20 Principle: The secret to achieving more with less* (New York: Doubleday).

Lattimore, D. (2017) "On the sidelines: An athlete's perspective of injury recovery," *Sport and Exercise Psychology Review*, 13(2): 13–21.

Lindsay, P., Thomas, O., and Douglas, G. (2010) "A framework to explore and transform client-generated metaphors in applied sport psychology," *The Sport Psychologist*, 24: 97–112.

Marshall, S., and Paterson, L. (2017) *The Brave Athlete: Calm the f*ck down and rise to the occasion* (Boulder, CO: VeloPress).

Meeusen, R., Duclos, M., Gleeson, M., Rietjens, G., Steinacker, J., and Urhausen, A. (2006) "Prevention, diagnosis and treatment of the Overtraining Syndrome," *European Journal of Sport Science*, 6(1): 1–14.

Moen, F., Myhre, K., and Sandbakk, Ø. (2016) "Psychological determinants of burnout, illness and injury among junior athletes," *The Sport Journal*. http://thesportjournal.org/article/psychological-determinants-of-burnout-illness-and-injury-among-elite-junior-athletes [accessed June 2019].

Putukian, M. (2016) "The psychological response to injury in student athletes: A narrative review with a focus on mental health," *British Journal of Sports Medicine*, 50(3): 145-148.

Richardson, S. O., Andersen, M. B., and Morris, T. (2008) *Overtraining Athletes: Personal journeys in sport* (Champaign, IL: Human Kinetics).

Saffary, R., Chin, L. S., and Cantu, R. C. (2012) "From concussion to chronic traumatic encephalopathy: A review," *Journal of Clinical Sport Psychology*, 6: 351–362.

Samuel, R. D., Tenenbaum, G., Mangel, E., Virshuvski, R., Chen, T., and Badir, A. (2015) "Athletes' experiences of severe injuries as a career-change event," *Journal of Sport Psychology in Action*, 6: 99–120.

Sandberg, S., and Grant, A. (2017) *Option B: Facing adversity, building resilience, and finding joy* (New York: Alfred A. Knopf).

Sapolsky, R. M. (2004) *Why Zebras Don't Get Ulcers*, 3rd edition (New York: Holt Paperbacks).

Smith, R. E., Schutz, R. W., Smoll, F. L., and Ptacek, J. T. (1995) "Development and validation of a multidimensional measure of sport-specific psychological skills: The athletic coping skills inventory-28," *Journal of Sport and Exercise Psychology*, 17(4): 379–398.

Stewart, M. A. (1995) "Effective physician–patient communication and health outcomes: A review," *Canadian Medical Association Journal*, 152(9): 1423–1433.

Taylor, J., and Taylor, S. (1997) *Psychological Approaches to Sports Injury Rehabilitation* (Philadelphia: Lippincott Williams & Wilkins).

Tracey, J. (2003) "The emotional response to the injury and rehabilitation process," *Journal of Applied Sport Psychology*, 15(4): 279–293.

Zimbardo, P., and Boyd, J. (2009) *The Time Paradox: The new psychology of time that will change your life* (New York: Free Press).

Zolli, A., and Healy, A. M. (2013) *Resilience: Why things bounce back* (New York: Simon & Schuster).

INDEX